All about A.D.D.

All about A.D.D.

Understanding Attention Deficit Disorder

Mark Selikowitz

Melbourne

OXFORD UNIVERSITY PRESS

Oxford   Auckland   New York

OXFORD UNIVERSITY PRESS AUSTRALIA
Oxford New York
Athens Auckland Bangkok Bombay
Calcutta Cape Town Dar es Salaam Delhi
Florence Hong Kong Istanbul Karachi
Kuala Lumpur Madras Madrid Melbourne
Mexico City Nairobi Paris Port Moresby
Singapore Taipei Tokyo Toronto
and associated companies in
Berlin Ibadan

OXFORD is a trade mark of Oxford University Press

National Library of Australia
Cataloguing-in-publication data:

Selikowitz, mark.
    All about ADD: understanding attention deficit disorder.

    Bibliography.
    Includes index.
    ISBN 0 19 553684 3.

    1. Attention-deficit hyperactivity disorder. 2. Attention-deficit hyperactivity disorder—
    treatment. 3. Attention deficit disordered children. I. Title. II. Title: All about attention
    deficit disorder.

616.8589

Edited by Elaine Cochrane
Designed by R.T.J. Klinkhamer
Cover photograph from the Stock Directory
Typeset by Desktop Concepts P/L, Melbourne
Printed through Bookpac Production Services, Singapore
Published by Oxford University Press
253 Normanby Road, South Melbourne, Australia

Preface

Awareness of attention deficit disorder (ADD) has been growing among both parents and professionals over the last five years. Television programmes and newspaper and magazine articles increasingly deal with this common and important condition.

Despite this media coverage, ignorance about ADD is widespread. This book aims to help overcome such ignorance. It provides a practical overview of ADD for all those who, in the broadest sense of the term, care for children. It will interest parents, teachers, doctors, psychologists, and the many other professionals, such as speech therapists and occupational therapists, who come into regular contact with children who struggle to learn, or have difficulty behaving appropriately for their age.

But if this book merely provides information it will have only partially fulfilled its purpose. If children with ADD and their parents are to be helped, knowledge alone will not suffice; it is essential that attitudes to children with this 'hidden disability' change.

It is, therefore, my hope that this book will lead its readers to a reappraisal of the way we interpret the developmental difficulties that so many children in our community face.

Hopefully we will banish useless words, such as 'lazy', 'stupid', and 'naughty', in favour of alternatives that lead us to a deeper understanding of these children, of the difficulties they contend with, and of their special needs. We will also have to appreciate how stressful such children can be to live with, so that we can provide their parents with the support they need.

Section one and Sections three to six of the book cover ADD in a general way. These sections will interest all parents.

In Section two, each of the six chapters is devoted to a specific area of development, and parents can select those chapters that are relevant to their child's particular difficulties.

To avoid using the cumbersome 'he or she' when referring to the child with ADD, I have used 'he' in some sections and 'she' in others. All statements apply equally to both sexes unless otherwise specified.

I am grateful to the parents of David, Martine, Peter and Greg who let me quote from their stories.

I am also grateful to Mrs Lynn McShane, who rapidly and accurately typed the manuscript from my dictation.

Mr Peter Rose of Oxford University Press kindly provided encouragement through all stages of this book's preparation.

I am indebted to my friend and colleague, Dr Rory McCarthy, with whom I share the approach to the diagnosis and management of ADD that is reflected in this text. The book has benefited from the regular exchange of ideas that working with Rory makes possible.

The addresses in the appendix were kindly supplied by Mr Peter Stauffer.

Finally, I thank my wife, Jill, who proofread the first draft of the typescript and made many valuable comments and suggestions. Her perspective as a teacher and a parent has been of great value. This book is dedicated to her, and to my children Daniel and Anne, with love.

Contents

Introduction

one

What is ADD?

A tale of two children

Dear Doctor

I am writing this letter to you before the appointment because I always find it difficult to remember what I wanted to say when I am sitting in front of a doctor.

We are desperate about David [age 7 years]—you are our last resort! We have been to numerous doctors, psychologists and psychiatrists already. They all make us feel that we are the cause of David's problem. We are tired of being analysed —we just want help.

David has been difficult from the moment he was born. The first two of our children were easy babies; but David was irritable from the very beginning. He hardly slept as an infant. He walked earlier than our other two, and from the time he took his first steps at 9 months he has been on the go. As a toddler he was into everything and had to be watched all the time. We tried him on a 'hyperactivity diet', but it did not help. Now that he is older, he is not as active, but he still never seems to tire, except when he is sick. I feel guilty admitting that it is only when he is ill that I enjoy having him at home.

He is like a walking disaster. He takes risks all the time, he has broken his leg twice and has numerous scars. He acts without stopping to think of the consequences, and he never seems to learn from his mistakes.

He won't do as he is told and if we try to discipline him, he becomes abusive and even aggressive. We have tried 'time-out' [putting him in his room, when disobedient, to cool down], but he destroys his room so it is just not worth it. On two occasions he jumped out of his bedroom window and ran away.

Living with David is like walking on eggshells. The slightest frustration sets him off into a rage. But sometimes he will be aggressive for no apparent reason. For example, yesterday his brother was sitting watching television and David came into the room, walked up to him and kicked him—out of the blue! He seemed sorry after he had done it, but I can't understand why he does things like that.

Each morning I wake up and get out of bed with a feeling of trepidation waiting to see what kind of a mood he is in, and what sort of a day we can expect. But even if he is in a good mood, it can change quite suddenly as the least thing sets him off.

Today is Saturday, and this morning he seemed all right, but then when he found his favourite T-shirt was in the wash, he started nagging and wanted to take it off the washing-line and wear it while it was still wet. I could not get him to see reason and he went on nagging for over one hour. Later, when I turned my back, he took it off the line and put it on. When I tried to take it off him, he started kicking and screaming and I just had to leave him alone. He is now in his room sobbing and kicking the door—we are in for another terrible weekend!

School has been a disaster for David. After the first week his teacher called me in to tell me he was impossible to teach. He wanders about the classroom; he calls out in class; he is noisy and he disrupts other children; his books are terribly messy; his work is never completed. The worst thing is that he is very rude to the teachers. He is easily affronted and takes any attempt to discipline him as a personal insult. He always seems to be getting punished, but it does not help. Earlier this term he was suspended from school for a week for swearing at a teacher. I had to take off work to stay with him, but I think he actually enjoyed the punishment.

He does not get on with the other children in the playground. He is very bossy with them and is not prepared to compromise. He has now earned a reputation as a bully, and is ostracised by the other children. He seems to get into punch-ups every day. I am sure he starts most of these. He will take on children who are older and larger than himself, so he often comes off second best. He was suspended from school for a week last term for punching a boy. The punishment made no difference to David—he was in a fight on his first day back!

I don't want you to think that David is always bad. He can be sweet and loving, and often he shows he is genuinely sorry for what he has done. But it never lasts for long—with David, trouble is always around the corner. Most worrying to us now is that David seems to be becoming depressed about his difficulties. Over the last month he has started saying that he is 'dumb'. He often says, 'Mummy, I don't know what is wrong with me'. Twice he has said that he wants to kill himself. We are terribly worried.

Dear Doctor

Martine is now 13 years old and we are concerned about her school progress. She is well behaved and does not get into any trouble at school, or at home, and this is why we have left it so long before seeking help.

Martine's reports have always been full of comments such as 'Martine needs to concentrate more', 'Martine has good potential if she were not so easily distracted'.

Martine is a vague, dreamy sort of child. Often when you talk to her she seems to be in a world of her own. One teacher thought she may be hard of hearing, but we had this tested and her hearing is perfect.

When you give her an instruction with more than three parts, she loses track of what she has to do. Yesterday I asked her to go to her room and take the sheets off her bed and put them in the wash. Ten minutes later I went to her room to find her sitting on her bed. She genuinely did not remember what I had asked her to do.

Her memory seems so inconsistent. She can tell you in detail about what happened years ago. Last week she surprised us by recognising someone in a photo whom she had not seen for years—and telling us all about her visit to this person's house very accurately. Yet today she cannot remember the spelling list she knew yesterday.

She is terribly disorganised. She is always losing things. She has to phone her friend most afternoons to find out what homework she is supposed to do.

She is also clumsy. She is a terrible fidget—some bit of her is always squirming when she should be sitting still.

But her greatest difficulty is in concentrating on school work. She sits down to her homework with the best of intentions, but she can't seem to persist with it. She is up and down at her desk and unless I sit with her nothing gets done. Even then it is a constant battle so that the whole family is upset. Getting her to complete assignments for school is impossible unless I do almost the whole thing for her. Her poor concentration is a problem at school as well. Her teachers complain that when all the other children have their eyes glued to their work, Martine is gazing out the window. Her work is often incomplete.

Martine says that she would like to become a teacher when she is an adult. We feel she is a clever girl, but if she continues like this, we can't see her achieving anything. Do you think you could help her?

David and Martine both came to see me. My assessments showed that they both had attention deficit disorder (ADD), and they were both greatly helped by treatment for this condition.

David has the form we call 'attention deficit disorder with hyperactivity' (ADD+H), while Martine has the form called 'attention deficit disorder without hyperactivity' (ADD–H). The conditions are very different, yet they are related to one another. They are like two sides of the same coin.

In neither form is the condition the parents' fault. Rather, it results from insufficient quantities of certain chemical messengers in the child's brain. The medicines used to treat ADD act by restoring these chemical messengers to more normal levels and so enable the child to behave and learn like other children. Careful diagnosis is essential to be certain that the child's difficulties are caused by ADD, and not by some other problem which may require different treatment.

The diagnosis, causes and treatment of ADD are discussed in the following chapters.

Overview of the features of ADD

All children with ADD have some features of the condition; *few will have all.* The features are listed in Table 1 and are outlined below.

Table 1   Features of ADD

Always present	May also be present
Poor concentration	Impulsivity
Task impersistence	Overactivity
Performance inconsistency	Social clumsiness
	Insatiability
	Disorganisation
	Inflexibility
	Clumsiness
	Learning difficulties
	Short-term memory problems
	Low self-esteem
	Defiant behaviour

Features that are always present

Poor concentration

Children with ADD cannot concentrate with the same ease as other children of the same age. The attentional mechanisms in their brains are still immature. This means that they have great difficulty concentrating on tedious tasks, such as school work, which greatly test these mechanisms.

Children with ADD have particular difficulties maintaining attention in a setting, such as a classroom, where there are many distractions. They do better in a one-to-one situation.

Children with ADD usually have much greater difficulty concentrating on things they have to listen to than things they have to look at. They have such difficulty listening that they can appear to have a problem hearing.

In milder cases, the child will be able to maintain attention for highly motivating and interactive activities, such as video games, and may be able to concentrate on tedious tasks, such as school work, for short periods. However, their immature concentrating mechanisms soon fatigue and their attention falters. The work of such children may be full of good beginnings and poor endings. They may be able to manage relatively well in the first part of the school day, but their performance usually falls off markedly in the second half.

Children with severe ADD may have difficulty staying on *any* task for very long, and may be unable to sit and watch a movie or play a game they enjoy. Such a child may constantly flit from one activity to another.

Poor concentration in children with ADD is described in more detail in the next chapter.

Impersistence

A common complaint is that children with ADD do not complete tasks.

At home parents find that they need to supervise their children more closely than do other parents with children of the same age. Simple chores, like getting dressed in the morning, take a long time. Parents often report that 'Nothing would get done if I was not on my child's back all the time'.

Children with ADD often forget what they are asked to do. Their parents may find them staring into space, or doing something quite different.

Impersistence is a particular problem with school work, as children with ADD often do not finish their set work. They may gaze out of the window, do something else, or start disrupting other children. As they get into high school and examinations become more important, this impersistence can seriously affect academic results, as children with ADD may not complete their examination papers.

Inconsistency

All children show some inconsistency in their performance, but this is particularly marked in children with ADD. With a tremendous amount of effort, children with ADD can sometimes concentrate and manage like other children, but they cannot maintain this effort most of the time.

It is this performance inconsistency that has so confused observers and led to many children with ADD being labelled as 'lazy' or 'naughty'. Those who do not understand the nature of ADD think that because a child performs appropriately on certain occasions, she is simply not trying hard enough when she fails. In the words of one psychiatrist, 'A child with ADD does well once and we hold that against him for the rest of his school career!'

Some situations make it easier for the child with ADD. The child may do well with close supervision in a one-to-one setting, in a novel situation, or with someone he or she is afraid of. Even in these situations, improved performance will not last and the old difficulties resurface.

Features that may also be present

Impulsivity

Children with ADD have great difficulty stopping to think before they act. (As Dennis the Menace said, 'By the time I think about it, I have done it!') Children with ADD often do the first thing that comes into their heads; they will blurt out answers in class; they may say tactless things; they may take many risks; they have tremendous difficulty waiting their turn. They are the sort of children who may run out in front of a car without looking first.

Because of this impulsivity they do not learn from their mistakes. The problem is not necessarily that children with ADD do not know the correct thing to do. They will often be able to explain in great detail what they should have done. They may also be quick to notice when others break the rules that they themselves do not obey. Nor is the problem that they do not want to do the right thing. They may be very upset and apologetic after the event. Their difficulty is in their lack of self-control.

The mechanisms that control behaviour in the brain seem to be immature and unreliable in the child with ADD. ADD is a problem of performance, not of knowledge. As Dr Russell Barclay, one of the foremost experts on this condition, put it: 'ADD is not a matter of not knowing what to do, but of not being able to do what you know.'

Impulsivity in children with ADD is discussed further in chapter 3.

Overactivity

Some children with ADD are continually on the go. The may be so restless as to seem to be 'driven by a motor'. Such a child often cannot remain seated, even for a few moments. He may wander around the classroom and the teacher may have great difficulty keeping him on his chair. Even when seated, some part of him may always be moving.

In the past, such overactivity (also known as hyperactivity) was considered an essential feature of ADD. We now know that while most children with ADD are more fidgety or restless than other children when carefully observed, many children with ADD are not overactive.

Even those who are very active when young may become less active than their peers as they get older—a transformation that has been described as changing from being a 'flipper' to a 'flopper' (in the sense of continually flopping down in front of the TV).

Overactivity in ADD is discussed in chapter 4.

Social clumsiness

Children with ADD often have difficulties reading social situations. They are often 'socially tone deaf'. They do not mean harm, but have a tendency to say very tactless things without realising the effect they are having. They seem to have difficulty predicting the consequences of their actions and responding appropriately to the occasion. They may 'come on too strong'. These children often do not pick up the same cues as other children of the same age. They often do not read facial expressions and may be oblivious to whether someone is angry or upset with them. Because they fail to develop the same degree of reserve as normal children, they may behave in front of others in ways that are not appropriate for children their age.

Although such abnormal behaviour may be apparent to all who meet the child, the people who are most likely to notice are the child's peers. With them, the child with ADD often sticks out like a sore thumb. Typically such children have little or no insight into how differently they are perceived. They do not seem to be able to learn the skills that are required to mix with others. They often become loners, or play with children younger or older than themselves. With younger children, they blend in because of their immaturity. With older children, more allowances are made for their inappropriate behaviour.

Social clumsiness in children with ADD is further described in chapter 6.

Insatiability

Children with ADD may be insatiable in their activities; not knowing when to stop, the way another child of their age would. This may be seen when they become overexcited in play and cannot calm down again when it is time to be serious.

Instead they become more and more excited and non-compliant. They may even become excessively defiant and provocative despite reasonable requests to calm down.

They may show their insatiability by never being satisfied with any treat and in nagging for more and more of things they want. This difficulty is related to problems that these children have with delaying gratification—they find it very difficult to wait for a reward or treat. Many parents find this insatiability the hardest part of ADD to manage.

Disorganisation

Many parents find that their child with ADD is continually losing things. Children with ADD find it very difficult to follow sequences without a great deal of supervision. When such supervision is not available, they become muddled and disorganised. Homework is forgotten at school, pens are misplaced, and possessions lost.

Inflexibility

Children with ADD are often very literal, and 'black and white' in their understanding of the world around them. They find it difficult to compromise. As a result parents often find themselves in conflict with their child over many issues.

'Every discussion is an argument' is a phrase parents often use to describe their child's behaviour. Once the child with ADD takes up an attitude to something, it is often almost impossible to get him or her to change. Children with ADD may become very fixated on certain rules and follow these rigidly. They have difficulty understanding when such rules can be reasonably bent.

Clumsiness

While some children with ADD are excellent athletes, most are poorly coordinated. Catching a small ball and writing neatly are skills which many children with ADD find extremely difficult. Many have low muscle tone (slight floppiness) when younger and have a poorly co-ordinated running style.

Learning difficulties

All children with ADD under-achieve academically. Most children with ADD will have difficulties in primary school with skills such as reading, spelling, and mathematics. Many have very untidy handwriting. Other common areas of difficulty are in reading comprehension and written expression.

Some children with mild ADD may do well during primary school. However, during high school such children often start to fall behind because greater skills in concentration and organisation are required.

Short-term memory problems

'An excellent memory for what happened last year, but she cannot remember what happened yesterday', is a common description of the child with ADD. Many know their multiplication or spelling list immediately after it has been taught, but cannot recall it the next day. Surprisingly, they often remember in great detail events that happened a long time ago.

Such children may have difficulty following an instruction with more than one part, becoming distracted or lost midway through carrying it out.

Poor incentival motivation

'Incentival motivation' refers to the ability to work for future rewards. As children grow older they have to defer gratification and be prepared to work for some future reward. Children with ADD find it very difficult to sacrifice now for a deferred reward. For example, they find it difficult to put in regular hours of study for something as intangible as good marks on a report card at the end of the year. They are very easily diverted from such study by the immediate gratification offered by watching TV or playing video games. This difficulty is a fundamental problem for many children with ADD.

Low self-esteem

Children with ADD are very hard on themselves. They may say negative things about themselves such as 'I am dumb!'. They may be tearful and easily hurt. They may feel dissatisfied with themselves even when they succeed. For example, a child with ADD who hit a cricket ball with great power complained that his father had bowled it too 'softly' to him. Some children with ADD who have low self-esteem may hide this behind bravado, bragging about themselves and putting down others as a way of managing their inferiority complex.

Poor self-esteem in ADD and the different types of behaviour it may give rise to are discussed in chapter 7.

Sleep problems

Many children with ADD have difficulty falling asleep and are up until late at night. Once asleep they may be very restless—their beds often look like a battlefield the next morning. Others may so exhaust themselves with their overactivity during the day that they fall asleep and sleep very soundly. Many children with ADD persist with bed-wetting later than other children. Night terrors, sleep walking, and bed-wetting are all more common in children with ADD.

Defiant behaviour

Many children with ADD have great difficulty obeying reasonable rules and regulations. When asked to do something by an authority figure they may refuse or even become abusive. Punishment often does not help. Children with ADD with defiant behaviour are very hard to discipline. As they get older they may get into problems with stealing, fire-lighting, and other anti-social behaviour.

Defiant behaviour is described further in chapter 5.

How common is ADD?

ADD is one of the most common conditions in childhood, affecting as many as 5 per cent of school-aged children. It affects about three times as many boys as girls and occurs in all ethnic groups.

It seems that boys with ADD are much more likely to be noticed than girls. While ADD is three times more common in boys in the community, many clinics see six times as many boys with the condition as girls. Nevertheless, ADD can be just as severe in a girl as a boy.

Historical background

- ADD is not a new condition. The first description of children with ADD was by an English physician, Dr George Still, in 1902. He described 20 children in his practice with impaired attention and overactivity.

  Interest in ADD was rekindled after an encephalitis epidemic in the USA in 1917–18. Many children acquired a form of encephalitis that left them with attention difficulties, overactivity, and impulsivity—features of ADD. In such children, the encephalitis virus had damaged parts of the brain that are probably immature in children with ADD, and hence their problems were similar.

  In the 1950s attention was focused on children with hyperactivity and the term 'hyperkinetic impulse disorder' was used. In the sixties the term 'minimal brain damage' was widely used for children with ADD.

  In the late sixties, attitudes to ADD in the UK and the USA began to diverge. In the UK, the term 'hyperactivity' was retained and only applied to children with severe overactivity. In the USA, a more subtle understanding of children with attention difficulties arose. First the term ADD was used, then later ADHD (attention deficit hyperactivity disorder) to encompass the spectrum of children with and without hyperactivity. Australia has increasingly followed the American view of ADD and has benefited from the huge amount of research undertaken in the USA, as well as the large amount of literature, videos, and equipment produced in the USA to help parents and teachers assist children with ADD.

  With the realisation that a proportion of children with ADD continue to have difficulties throughout adulthood, an increasing amount of literature is now being devoted to residual ADD in adults.

Summary points

- ADD occurs in two forms—with overactivity, and without.
- All children with ADD have some of the features of the condition; few will have all.
- Features that are always present are:
  Poor concentration
  Task impersistence
  Performance inconsistency
- Features that may also be present are:
  Impulsivity
  Overactivity
  Social clumsiness
  Insatiability
  Disorganisation
  Inflexibility
  Clumsiness
  Learning difficulties
  Short-term memory problems
  Low self-esteem
  Sleep problems
  Defiant behaviour
- ADD affects 5% of school age children. It affects both boys and girls, but is three times more common in boys.
- ADD is not a new condition, but our understanding of this condition has increased greatly over the last two decades. ADD is now more likely to be picked up early and treated effectively.

Some characteristic difficulties

two

Poor concentration

'Peter must pay attention.' 'Peter is too easily distracted in class.' 'Peter must take care not to be so careless.' These are the comments that keep recurring in our son's report cards from year to year. It has always been difficult to get Peter to concentrate on school work. His mind always seems to be elsewhere. When he does attend, he is soon distracted. Getting him to do his homework is a constant battle. Last year I was finding it so stressful, that I decided not to get involved with his homework at all. As a result, Peter spent many afternoons on detention. Unfortunately, this did not seem to help.

Peter's distracted state means that he often does not hear what the teacher is saying. He often loses notes that he should bring home.

He has trouble carrying out instructions at home too. If I ask him to do something he gets distracted mid-way through, or forgets what I asked him to do.

He is terribly disorganised. I have to organise and supervise him in everything. If I did not keep tabs on everything he needs to do for school he would never succeed. In the last three weeks he has lost his glasses, his school diary, and his lunch box.

The perplexing thing is that Peter can concentrate very well when something interests him. He can spend hours totally fixated on a video game. When I pointed this out to my family doctor he thought that it meant that Peter did not have ADD. But the assessment by the paediatrician and psychologist showed that Peter does have ADD and the effect of the medicine has been remarkable.

Poor concentration in children with ADD

Children with ADD often have difficulty giving close attention to details. As a result they make careless mistakes in their school work. They often do not follow through on instructions and fail to finish school work, chores, and other duties. Children with ADD are very easily distracted, particularly in a group setting. They tend to be forgetful in daily activities. Their difficulties seem to be greater for concentration on things they have to listen to (auditory attention) than things they have to look at (visual attention).

To understand the difficulties that children with ADD face we must first understand the attentional process in the brain.

The attentional process in the brain

When we look at something, a great deal of information about everything in our field of vision travels from our eyes to the brain. This picture of our whole visual field is known as the *visual buffer*. Our brain is able to select a portion of this information to focus on. This portion selected for attention is called the *attentional window*.

The attentional window can be shifted voluntarily from one part of the visual buffer to another. Not only can it change its location, but it can also expand or shrink its scope, like a zoom lens. That is, from all the visual information entering the brain, we select what we will pay attention to and how closely we will pay attention, and we can change this at will. With an efficient attentional mechanism in the brain, the attentional window can be focused on one part of the visual buffer for long periods of time.

The efficiency with which attention can be sustained increases as children grow older.

A younger child's attention will wander unless the material in the attentional window is very interesting and the information in the rest of the visual buffer is relatively boring. Even then, the attentional mechanisms quickly tire and attention cannot be sustained for long.

There is a comparable attentional mechanism for listening. The *auditory buffer* contains all the sounds heard at a particular time. The *auditory attention window* focuses on one particular source of sound, in the way a radio tunes into one particular frequency. Selecting part of the buffer and sustaining attention on one part of it is generally more difficult for auditory than for visual stimuli—listening is generally harder than looking. This is especially so for children with ADD.

Difficult tasks for attentional mechanisms

Although children with ADD have immature attentional mechanisms that quickly tire, it is wrong to believe that children with ADD cannot concentrate at all. Their mechanisms for concentrating are inefficient and unreliable, not absent. It is this that makes their performance so inconsistent.

Having an immature concentrating mechanism is like having a weak leg that allows one to walk for short bursts, but does not allow one to keep up with one's peers for long stretches. Children with ADD are easily fatigued when their attention needs to be sustained

Attentional mechanisms are more stressed under certain circumstances than others, and it is in the difficult situations that children with ADD are most likely to find that their attentional mechanisms are failing.

Tedious tasks are very difficult for immature attentional mechanisms. This is why younger children cannot be expected to concentrate on tedious tasks. Unfortunately much of the work that school children need to perform is very tedious and children with ADD quickly become distracted. It is not that a normal child finds the work any more interesting than the child with ADD, it is just that the normal child finds concentrating easier.

The attentional difficulties may give children with ADD an unfocused appearance. Common descriptions include 'vague', 'dreamy', and having 'glazed eyes'.

Because children with ADD tire easily when having to concentrate, their work may be full of good beginnings which then peter out. Often their school work will be much better in the morning when they are fresher and better able to compensate for their attentional difficulties. This may be true for all children, but for those with ADD the contrast will be greater.

If the task is long or arduous, children with ADD quickly lose concentration. This is why they are so often described as being impersistent. This is further compounded by their difficulty in working for a distant reward—their lack of incentival motivation.

Difficulties with concentration also result in children with ADD often being confused and unable to understand instructions. When the child with ADD has to listen, he has difficulty remaining tuned to the 'right station'. His concentration is easily distracted onto other sounds and so he hears only parts of the instruction. No wonder parents say that their instructions go in one ear and out the other. These difficulties may be compounded by the problems with short-term memory and language comprehension that frequently occur in children with ADD.

A common observation made about the visual attention of children with ADD is that they may seem to 'see everything at a glance'. Because of their difficulty with sustained attention, they may become reliant on a quick appraisal of any new situation. They may, therefore, surprise parents and teachers by how much they can take in with seemingly little effort. However, they have difficulty absorbing more than the superficial features.

Children with ADD tend to flit from one thing to another. Parents often notice how poor such children are at occupying themselves. Having moved quickly from one toy, or activity, to another, they quickly lose concentration and can then become aimless. It is at times like these that their behaviour may become attention seeking, or that they may get into mischief.

Another difficulty for children with ADD is in adjusting their level of attention to suit the situation. For example, children may be less focused in the playground and then need to become more attentive when they return to the classroom after recess. Children with ADD have great difficulty coping with such transitions. Instead of increasing their state of alertness once in the classroom, like other children of the same age, they remain unfocused and do not settle back to work again.

Children with ADD have their greatest difficulty sustaining concentration if there are many distractions. The usual classroom is full of distractions because of the presence of so many other children, and children with ADD are at their worst in such an environment. By contrast, they are at their most attentive and learn best in a one-to-one setting.

Sometimes a small group of children with ADD is withdrawn from the large classroom for special help, in the hope that they will do better with fewer distractions. However, this environment is likely to be very distracting because children with ADD usually distract one another. Whenever possible, children with ADD should not be grouped together in a class.

Children with ADD will concentrate best if they are receiving frequent positive feedback. They usually manage best if the work is very interesting and if there are immediate consequences for their actions.

Their concentration is usually at its best early in the day and diminishes as their attentional mechanisms fatigue. Parents and teachers are advised to arrange for demanding work to be done in the first part of the day, and to make some allowance for reduced concentration as the day progresses.

Noisiness and attention in ADD

Research has shown that as children with ADD concentrate more intently, they become noisier. It seems as if they need to provide some constant noise and self-talk to focus on a task. This can easily be misinterpreted by a teacher who believes the child is becoming noisier because she is not working, rather than because she *is* working. Allowances should be made for such productive, involuntary noisiness.

Summary points

- Children with ADD usually have greater problems with auditory than visual attention.
- Tedious tasks test attentional mechanisms the most.
- Performance inconsistency is the hallmark of an immature attentional mechanism.
- The attention of children with ADD quickly fatigues.
- Children with ADD may move quickly from one task to another and may lack self-direction. They often become bored quickly and may become disruptive and attention seeking.
- They are easily distracted in a classroom setting.
- Children with ADD have difficulty changing their level of attention during transitions from one setting to another.
- Paradoxically, they may become noisier when they are attending appropriately than when they are not.

three

Impulsivity

Impulsivity, the difficulty in being able to think before acting, causes many problems for children with ADD both at home and at school. The problem of impulsivity in a child with ADD is not solved by teaching the child to consider the consequences of an action. Children with this condition lack the reflective and behavioural inhibition mechanisms needed to apply such teaching to their everyday lives.

Behavioural inhibition mechanisms in the brain

Normal preschool children are impulsive creatures. If they see something they want, they usually cannot resist the temptation to take it. If they do not like something, they act out their aggression or frustration without any thought of the consequences. We regard this as normal behaviour at this age.

Jeffrey A. Gray first proposed the theory that certain structures in the frontal part of the brain act as a behavioural inhibition system (BIS) to control behaviour. Gray's theory was based on work with rat brains, but identical structures exist in the human brain. Some authorities believe that the reason very young children are so impulsive is that their brain BIS is not yet active. Their behaviour is like a simple reflex arc, like a knee jerk reaction.

As the frontal lobe of the brain develops, the nerve cells or neurones that control behaviour become more powerful and start playing a mediating role between the input and output of the brain. This allows the individual to stop and think before acting. Only then can the knowledge and experience which the child has acquired play a role in preventing impulsive responses.

Children with ADD who behave in an impulsive way do not do so because of ignorance. They usually know as well as other children of their age what they should and should not do. However, they respond in a reflexive (impulsive) way to the things that happen around them. If one observes the behaviour of a child with ADD with this in mind, their repeated misdemeanours and failure to 'learn' from their mistakes, and from punishment, is understandable.

Telling a child with ADD to 'stop and think' is often asking the impossible. It would be analogous to asking an adult not to put out a hand to break a fall. The knowledge that one is going to fall on something soft does not allow one to inhibit the reflex action of stretching out one's hands. Similarly, knowledge is not enough to stop the child with ADD from behaving impulsively. It is only when behaviour inhibition systems start to become active, either as a result of normal brain maturation, or by being 'switched on' by medication (as will be discussed in chapter 13), that the child with ADD is able to stop and think before acting.

Manifestations of impulsivity

The impulsivity of children with ADD manifests itself in many ways. They act impulsively, think impulsively, and feel things impulsively.

Most obvious is the tendency to act without thinking. This may mean that the child endangers herself or others by risk-taking acts. It also means that the child is likely to make heedless or careless errors because of her failure to think carefully.

Children with ADD will sometimes act on a whim or with minimal encouragement, especially from another child, and other children will take advantage of this. Children with ADD are often 'set up' by other children to do things that the other children recognise as dangerous. Their difficulties are further compounded because they generally lack the guile not to get caught. Often a child with ADD will join in with a number of other children in carrying out some misdemeanour, and only the child with ADD will be caught. A further disadvantage is that the child with ADD, having gained a reputation for fool-hardy behaviour, is often blamed for a misdemeanour whether guilty or not.

Because they take risks, children with ADD are very accident prone. It is common for children with ADD to have broken a number of bones during their childhood. Accidental poisoning and burning are also more common in this group of children.

Children with ADD are often compulsively destructive. They are quick to damage or destroy toys. Parents are often puzzled because their child may destroy toys that he enjoys. They do not seem to be able to control this behaviour. Their impulsivity also means that they are generally harder on their toys and are more likely to damage their parents' property and the property of others.

It is extremely difficult for an impulsive child to wait in line when queueing is needed. He is also likely to blurt out in class and to find it very difficult to wait his turn in a game or other activity.

Children who are impulsive quickly learn to take short cuts in the way in which they do things. They want to finish things very quickly and will find all kinds of ways of getting to the end of an activity without worrying about the quality of what they produce.

Impulsivity gets in the way of delaying gratification, and children with this difficulty find it almost impossible to work for a long-term goal. They are reward-driven like other children, but need that reward immediately. Parents will find that if a treat is promised, children with ADD will nag incessantly while waiting for it. Parents often learn not to tell their child about treats and outings because they want to avoid the constant nagging that goes on until the reward or treat is given, and because these children over-react should the outing or treat not transpire.

Children with ADD often cannot stop themselves from touching things or people. Other children of the same age often respond very badly to this touching. Parents often complain that children with ADD cannot keep their hands to themselves. The habit of touching things can be very embarrassing to the parents when they take their child out, and things may get broken when the child is visiting or shopping.

Verbal impulsivity makes children with ADD very illogical at times. Instead of thinking about things in a clear sequence, they move impulsively from one idea to another. It is very difficult to reason with a child who thinks in this way.

Situations or games requiring sharing, cooperation and restraint with peers are particularly problematical. Group situations are particularly difficult for children with ADD, because it is in such situations that the individual's impulsivity must be subjugated to the needs of the whole group.

A tendency towards impulsivity interferes with a child's ability to carry out sequential tasks, that is, the ability to get things into the right order. Children with significant difficulty in sequential organisation will experience problems with tasks such as following directions, counting, telling time, using a calendar and getting to know the day's schedule. Such a child will often have difficulty getting dressed quickly, having the correct books ready for a class, getting to the right classroom, and following complex instructions. It may also result in spelling errors such as 'hegde' for 'hedge' and 'fisrt' for 'first'.

This is why children with ADD often benefit from having a set routine, and are at their best in a structured situation where their impulsivity is contained. A regular course of events helps a child anticipate the next activity and remember the schedule.

Emotional impulsivity results in quick changes of mood. Children show this by having 'a short fuse' and a low frustration tolerance. Parents will notice that the child seems to be managing quite well and then suddenly becomes upset for no apparent reason.

Children with ADD may have difficulty controlling their impulse to be noisy. Generally they are boisterous children who are more talkative than their peers.

Management of impulsivity

Cognitive therapy, a form of therapy that aims to teach children self-control, has shown disappointing results in children with ADD. In contrast, medication can play a very dramatic role in controlling impulsivity. In many children medicine alone is enough to ameliorate this difficulty.

Parents, teachers and others who come into contact with the child with ADD need to understand that impulsive behaviour is not completely under the child's control. Wherever possible, allowances should be made for this. Environmental changes and modification of goals are important ways of helping the child. For example, parents should ensure that children with ADD who take risks because of their impulsivity are properly supervised in potentially dangerous situations. Matches, sharp knives, and other potentially dangerous implements may need to be kept out of the child's reach. Short-term, easily obtainable goals may need to be set. For example, it may be unrealistic to punish an impulsive child with ADD every time she calls out an answer in class. It may be more appropriate to set her the goal of not more than one such outburst per lesson. The child should be praised if she successfully limits her behaviour in this way.

Summary points

- Children with ADD who behave in an impulsive way do not do so because of ignorance. They usually know just as well as other children what they should and should not do.
- Children with ADD:
  act impulsively
  think impulsively
  experience emotions impulsively
- Consequences of impulsivity include:
  risk-taking
  compulsive destructiveness
  difficulty waiting for his turn
  taking short cuts
  touching people and things
  illogical reasoning
  difficulties with sequential organisation
  sudden temper outbursts
- Treatment of impulsivity includes:
  making allowances for the child's difficulty
  creating a consistent environment and a predictable routine
  medication

four

Overactivity

Greg was overactive even before he was born. When I was pregnant with him, I often could not get to sleep at night because he used to kick so much. He was fine as a young baby, but from about nine months, when he first learned to walk, he became a handful. We used the same cot for all four children, but only Greg was able to climb out by the time he was one year old. He would climb up onto tables, chairs, anywhere he could. He had no sense of danger. He seemed not to feel pain. He would fall down and simply get back up again. He did not understand the word 'No!'. He had to be watched every minute.

By the end of the day I was exhausted with continually supervising him. Then the battle would start to try to get him to sleep. He would still be up at midnight, his older brothers and his sister would be fast asleep by about 8.30. He could not be kept in his bedroom and would come into the lounge. He would be tired and unreasonable and climb all over my husband and me, but we could not get him to stay in bed.

He started at preschool when he was three and a half and the teacher complained that he was aggressive towards the other children. He also would not sit down during story-time or stay on his mattress during rest time. A special assistant was employed by the preschool to help Greg cope and things seemed to settle down.

When Greg was due to start school at five, the preschool teacher suggested that he was not mature enough and should stay on at the preschool for another year. During that year he settled down quite a lot and we thought he was ready for school.

The first year of proper school was a disaster for Greg. He spent most of the time being punished for getting out of his seat, for calling out, and for disrupting the other children. The other children called him a 'Naughty Greg' and he became more and more discouraged and defiant. He did not seem to be learning anything at school at all. He was always in trouble, and seemed to be blamed for everything, even though it sometimes was not his fault. At the end of the year the teacher told me that if she had to teach Greg for another year she would have resigned!

At the end of the first week of his second year at school, his new teacher sent a note home asking to see me. She said that Greg was impossible to teach. She suggested we take Greg to a paediatrician for an assessment because he seemed hyperactive and may need medication. This was the first time that medicine was suggested.

We had the assessment which showed that Greg was a very intelligent boy, but that he had ADD. We had never heard of this condition before. We read everything we could about the condition and after satisfying ourselves that the medication was perfectly safe, Greg was started on Ritalin [methylphenidate]. The change in his behaviour and mood was miraculous. One hour after the tablet I had my first proper conversation with Greg. For the first time in his life he was able to sit still and look at a book. He was able to sit down at mealtimes like the other children.

The teacher reported a wonderful change in Greg at school. All of a sudden his reading came along and his whole attitude to life changed. The other children started to be more positive about him and he was invited to his first birthday party.

Now five years later, Greg still takes Ritalin every day. If he forgets a tablet he gets into trouble at school because of his behaviour. He calls them his 'thinking tablets' and they have made all the difference to his life and ours.

Temporary immobilisation— a developmental skill

If one visits a preschool and observes a group of three year olds, and then visits a primary school and observes a group of eight year olds, one notices an important difference: the three year olds are more restless and fidgety than the eight year olds.

Filming of children of different ages shows that the level of activity in normal children decreases markedly in the first three years of life and then, more gradually, over the rest of the school years.

This is most likely to be due to the greater influence, with increasing age, of inhibiting mechanisms in the brain that temporarily immobilise parts of the body when they are not needed. Young children cannot efficiently immobilise muscles in this way and associated and 'mirror' movements of their bodies are common. 'Mirror' movements occur when a child does something with one part of the body and another part moves in unison. Younger children also have more 'overflow' movements, a tendency for some parts of the body to move when the child is excited or concentrating (e.g. moving the tongue while writing).

The persistence of immaturities of motor function, such as mirror movements and overflow phenomena, constitute part of the 'soft' neurological signs that are common in children with ADD of all ages and provide evidence of immaturity of parts of the brain that control movement in these children.

Many children with ADD continue to have a degree of muscular overactivity that indicates that movement inhibiting mechanisms in the brain do not seem to be as mature as they should be.

These movement inhibition mechanisms are not under voluntary control, although with great effort a child can temporarily over-ride them. This cannot be sustained for long however. Asking a child with ADD and hyperactivity to sit still is asking the impossible.

Varying degrees of overactivity

No aspect of ADD has caused more confusion than that of overactivity. As discussed in the first chapter, ADD used to be called 'hyperactivity'. This meant that unless overactivity was present, the diagnosis was not made. However, we now know that overactivity may be so mild as to go unnoticed in children with the disorder.

The degree of overactivity of children with ADD varies from the child with nothing more than excessive feelings of restlessness, to the child who is almost never still.

There are no instruments that reliably measure activity levels.

Three descriptive catogories of overactivity are usually recognised.

I.   Restless feelings

Many children with ADD are not unusually active for their age, but simply complain of feelings of restlessness.

II.   'Fidgets'

A child with the 'fidgets' may be described as 'a can of worms', 'a rocker', 'a jiggler', 'a wriggler', or 'a squirmer'. These children may squirm their bodies when they are seated. They may fidget with their hands, for example by drumming on the table or fiddling with things on their desk.

III.   'Runners and climbers'

Children with ADD who have the more severe form of overactivity are often described as 'being driven by a motor'. Such children are almost never still. They run instead of walking. They do not like to be restricted in any way. If held, they usually try to wriggle free. They will clamber over objects and climb onto things when other children of their age no longer do such things.

Such behaviour often leads to repeated falls and injuries such as bruises, cuts, and grazes. This is particularly the case because children with ADD often have a poor sense of danger, are impulsive, and learn poorly from experience.

When children with this sort of overactivity level become tired, their activity level often increases instead of decreasing, making it difficult for them to fall asleep.

Under-activity in older children

Most overactive children with ADD become less active as they get older. Some remain 'outdoor' children who much prefer being active to sitting still. Some may develop normal levels of activity as adolescents.

Other children with ADD may become less active than their non-ADD peers in adolescence. These children become reluctant to take part in physical activities. They prefer to spend time in front of the television or video game. Such 'couch potatoes' run the risk of becoming obese from eating inappropriately for their activity level.

Summary points

- Children with ADD who have overactivity resemble younger children in relation to movement inhibition mechanisms in the brain. They can inhibit their overactivity for only very short periods.
- Overactivity in children with ADD can be classified according to the degree of severity:
  I   Feelings of restlessness only
  II 'Fidgets'
  III 'Runners and climbers'
- Some children with ADD may be under-active from the start, others may become under-active in adolescence.

five

Defiance

Approximately one quarter of children with ADD experience significant difficulties conforming to the rules and regulations appropriate for their age. These difficulties are usually seen both at home and at school, although some children can cope with a very structured situation at school and experience all their difficulties in the home setting.

This defiant behaviour is often misunderstood by observers who think that there must be something wrong with the way that the parents are disciplining their child.

Parents of such children often report that their friends, as well as strangers, will make suggestions, such as 'you are not being tough enough', or 'if you gave her a good hiding she would stop doing that'. Unfortunately the management of defiant behaviour in children with ADD is not so simple.

Compliance—a function of the brain

Normal toddlers have great difficulty complying with their parents' instructions. The phrase 'terrible twos' is widely used to describe the great difficulty that children have between the ages of about 15 months and 3 years in obeying parental commands. At that stage of development, the brain is simply not mature enough to allow the child to inhibit self-centred needs, to delay gratification, and to conform. At that stage the brain has not yet developed its mechanism that we generally call 'conscience'. Children of that age are not yet able to put themselves into someone else's place and to understand how their behaviour is affecting others. They simply act out their feelings and do the things they feel they want to do, without regard to the consequences.

As the brain develops, this lawlessness is inhibited by the increasing activity of the frontal lobe. It has been known for a long time that adults who sustain damage to certain parts of the brain can start behaving in a defiant, non-compliant manner (just like 'terrible twos').

In many children with ADD, the necessary mechanisms for compliance with rules and regulations develop slowly. This means that although the child is in an ordinary home and ordinary school, he cannot conform like other children of his age.

Our society has great difficulty accepting this. We feel uncomfortable with the idea that children who are behaving poorly may be doing so because of a brain disorder. We like to have someone to blame for the child's difficulties and we focus on the child's parents.

In fact, children with ADD with non-compliant behaviour have parents who are just as competent as other parents. They are usually at their wit's end to know what to do with their extremely difficult child. Many have experience of raising children without behaviour problems, only to give birth to a child with ADD who does not respond to the usual methods of discipline.

Parents of such children quickly learn that smacking and other forms of punishment are ineffective. They are therefore forced into passive acceptance of much unwanted behaviour, which only seems to confirm the casual observer's view that they are being too lenient. Such observers often do not realise that the parents have been forced to become lenient because other strategies have failed. If they were to smack their child, or use 'time out', whenever she perpetrated a misdemeanour, they would be forced to smack the child continually, or she would have to spend most of her waking hours locked in her room.

Another aspect of such children's behaviour is its variability. This also leads to misunderstanding. For example, an 8 year old with ADD who has the compliance of a two year old will be very inconsistent in the way in which he behaves in different situations. This is why parents often use the term 'Jekyll and Hyde' to describe their child. It is not simply that the child is never compliant. At certain times, for example when he is not tired or when he tries extremely hard, he will be successful in behaving well. However, he cannot maintain this for protracted periods of time, or in all the situations that a child of his age should be able to. Sometimes he will be better with one parent, usually the father. This may be because he is less familiar with his father, or because the father is quicker to resort to painful physical discipline.

Unfortunately, such performance inconsistency, which is a prominent feature of ADD, is often misinterpreted as implying that the child could succeed if only he tried. This is analogous to saying that because a child with heart disease can walk 15 metres without becoming breathless, he should be able to run a marathon, if only he tried hard enough. It is the difficulty with *sustained* performance that shows up the problems of the child with ADD, in the same way as it does for the child with heart disease. Sustained performance is the true test of the competence and maturity of the brain functions that are impaired in children with ADD.

Observers may think that children with ADD should be able to comply with rules because they know and understand them. But ADD is a *performance* disability, not a *knowledge* disability. Children with ADD usually know what they should do and should not do; they simply cannot consistently do the things that they know they should.

Severity of defiant behaviour

Non-compliant behaviour in children with ADD can be divided into two forms. The more common, milder form, is known as *oppositional disorder*, while the more severe, fortunately more rare, form is known as *conduct disorder*.

Oppositional disorder

Approximately one quarter of all children with ADD have oppositional behaviour. Such children demonstrate several of the following behaviours:

Active defiance

Children with oppositional disorder will flout rules. They often refuse to do their homework, to carry out household chores, or to conform to requests such as wearing a complete school uniform. Any child without ADD may defy adult instructions, but children with oppositional behaviour do this in a far more extreme way, persisting despite repeated punishment.

Argumentativeness

Parents will often say that, with the child who has oppositional behaviour, 'every discussion is an argument'. Often the only communication between parent and child is in the form of arguments. Children with oppositional behaviour will characteristically argue with all adults, including teachers and even strangers, in a way that other children of the same age would not do.

Temper outbursts

Children with oppositional disorder have temper tantrums of the kind that are usually not seen in school-age children. They resemble the tantrums seen in toddlers.

Often parents will report that their child will be reasonable until any of his desires are thwarted or frustrated in any way. He will then suddenly have a temper tantrum, kicking walls, slamming doors and shouting. If put in his room for 'time out' (see chapter 12) he may totally destroy his possessions. Some will even escape through the window.

The temper tantrums may be so sudden, and so out of proportion to what has happened, that parents may think the child is having some form of seizure. An unusual form of epilepsy (temporal lobe epilepsy) does have to be considered in any child who has unprovoked temper outbursts; however, in children with oppositional disorder it is not that the temper tantrum is unprovoked, it is simply that the trigger is so insignificant.

Deliberately annoying and provoking other individuals

Children with oppositional disorder tend to interfere with others. They seem to be unable to resist the temptation to provoke other children. Often they cannot go past a sibling without punching him or her. In the playground, teachers may notice that the child with oppositional disorder will grab another child's possessions and run off with them so as to provoke him or her. Such children often have no understanding of their own vulnerability and will provoke children who are much larger than themselves without realising the consequences.

'Touchiness'

Children with oppositional behaviour are extremely easily annoyed. They will be slighted by the most minor action and then will become very angry and aggressive. Once more, it is the frequency and severity of these outbursts that distinguish them from the normal child.

Projection of blame

Children with oppositional behaviour tend to blame others for their own inadequacies. Any mistake on their part is immediately attributed to someone else such as a parent, a teacher, or a friend.

Resentfulness

Children with oppositional disorder often deeply resent any authority figure. They will therefore complain bitterly about anyone who tries to discipline them. They may be quick to develop a deep hatred for any authority figures they come across.

Spitefulness and vindictiveness

These are characteristics often seen in children with oppositional behaviour. For no apparent reason, they will try to hurt another person. It is usually siblings who suffer the most from this sort of behaviour, but sometimes parents will notice that a child with oppositional behaviour will behave spitefully towards a younger child on first meeting. They may be very cruel to children who are weak or vulnerable in some way.

They tend to bear grudges and will seek revenge long after any real or imagined misdemeanour against them.

Swearing

Even from an early age, children with oppositional behaviour are quick to learn swear words. They will often use obscene language in a situation where a child of their age would know that this is not appropriate. The best way to handle swearing is to ignore it, but this often does not resolve the problem in these children.

Conduct disorder

Conduct disorder is more severe than oppositional disorder and occurs in about 5 per cent of children with ADD. Conduct disorder differs from oppositional disorder in that the problems attract a greater degree of social disapproval, and often result in the child breaking the law.

Some children will develop conduct disorder at an early age, even as early as 7 or 8 years. Most, however, start off with oppositional disorder and then develop conduct disorder in the teenage years. Most are male.

Some children with conduct disorder are the 'solitary aggressive' type. These children are loners and carry out their offences on their own. More common are the 'group type offenders', who are attracted to other children with similar problems. Group type offenders may behave quite reasonably when on their own, but become anti-social when part of their group (gang).

The behaviours seen in children with conduct disorder include the following:

Stealing

Children with conduct disorder steal often and repeatedly. They may do this *without confrontation*, where possessions are taken when the owner is absent, or *with confrontation*, when they threaten the owner before removing the possession. Stealing with confrontation is of even greater concern than stealing without confrontation, because it may be accompanied by assault.

Running away

It is rare for children with conduct disorder not to have run away from home overnight on at least two occasions. Often this becomes a repeated pattern of behaviour and parents may not know where their children are for long stretches of time.

Repeated lying

Normal children may lie in order to avoid punishment. Children with oppositional behaviour also lie in order to obtain something that they want. In fact, lying becomes so common that it becomes very difficult for parents to know when the child is telling the truth and when he is not.

Setting fires

Normal or oppositional children may play with matches on occasions. Children with conduct disorder are more persistent in the way in which they set fires. Rather than simply experimenting with matches, they will try to burn down buildings such as their school or home.

Truanting

Children with conduct disorder will spend a great deal of time wagging school (see School avoidance, chapter 7).

Breaking in

Breaking in to a house, a building, or a car is common in children with conduct disorder. This may be associated with stealing or joyriding, or may be an end in itself.

Destroying property

Children with oppositional disorder often have a compulsion to damage things. They may destroy their toys and other possessions.

Children with conduct disorder will often go about destroying other people's possessions. They may walk through the streets breaking windows and damaging cars. They often resent other people having possessions.

Spray-painting cars and walls is becoming an increasingly common behaviour among children with conduct disorder.

Physical cruelty to animals

Children with conduct disorder often lack the compassion towards animals that is usually seen in children. They seem to enjoy taking advantage of animals' vulnerability, and parents will sometimes become aware that their child is becoming cruel in the way in which he treats pets and other neighbourhood animals. On occasion, children with conduct disorder have behaved cruelly towards animals in zoos and wildlife parks.

Forcing sexual activity

Forcing sexual activity is more common in the 'group type' of child with conduct disorder. The victims are usually female.

Using weapons

Many children with conduct disorder are fascinated by weapons. They may start collecting knives and even firearms. Some will try to use these.

Initiating fights

Children with conduct disorder seem to enjoy getting into fights. They may regularly come home having been involved in some altercation. These may be with other groups or with individuals.

The characteristic of children with conduct disorder is that they initiate fights and seek out confrontation.

Physical cruelty to people

Younger siblings are often the first victims of this form of violence. While it is quite normal for siblings to argue and fight, the behaviour of children with conduct disorder is characterised by the degree of cruelty shown towards younger siblings.

A younger sibling is in a very vulnerable situation. The younger child cannot physically defend herself from the older, stronger individual with whom she must share the home. Often the older sibling will wait until the parents' backs are turned and then do all he can to batter the sibling.

Little attention has been directed towards 'sibling abuse', or 'domestic violence against siblings'. Some siblings are assaulted in a way that would result in legal proceedings if this had not occurred within the home. Parents have a responsibility towards the younger sibling to ensure that he or she is not subjected to such treatment.

Treatment of defiant behaviour

Oppositional disorder

Mild oppositional behaviour will often resolve with medication alone. Once a child is on appropriate medication for ADD, she usually becomes calmer and her behaviour more compliant. Aggression also decreases.

It is helpful if parents also learn behaviour management techniques so that they can implement these together with the medical treatment (see chapter 12).

For children with more severe oppositional disorder, behaviour management needs to be looked at in greater detail. In such cases, it is important that a psychologist is involved to provide parents with appropriate strategies for managing their child's behaviour. These, used in conjunction with medication, will not totally eradicate the behaviours, but will ensure that the child is more manageable and is less likely to do harm to himself or others. It also makes the later development of conduct disorder less likely.

Conduct disorder

Management of conduct disorder is extremely difficult. There are some children with conduct disorder who will respond positively to medication, so medication should always be tried. Unfortunately, medication does not help many children with conduct disorder. Even in those children where medication is helpful, it can be extremely difficult to get the child to take it consistently. Such children often deny that the medication helps them, even when it is quite clear to parents and other observers that it does! Parents may need to exert a lot of energy in order to ensure that medicine is taken.

Children with conduct disorder often experiment with alcohol and marijuana and parents often wonder whether medicines used for ADD will interact with these. Medicines that are used in ADD do not interact in any adverse way with alcohol or marijuana. However, marijuana and alcohol tend to make children poorly motivated and lacking in inhibition, while the medicines used for ADD make them better focused and motivated. Marijuana and alcohol therefore undermine the effect of the medicine.

It is important that parents of a child with conduct disorder receive counselling to help them develop strategies for coping with their child's behaviour. Most parents will need someone outside the family to talk to about their concerns, and to look at different ways of dealing with their child's behaviour.

Parents of a child with conduct disorder are in an extremely difficult situation. They want to keep the child out of trouble, but the child often seems bent on a course of self-destruction. All that parents can do is to try to be available when their child needs them, and hope that with time the brain will mature and the behaviour settle.

There certainly are no easy answers to questions about the appropriateness of special school units or special residential units for children with conduct disorder. These issues need to be looked at on an individual basis. The decision about whether to involve the police can also be a difficult one when the child's aggression is directed towards parents or their property. If the child's behaviour is placing others at risk, the police may have to be involved.

Individual psychotherapy (counselling) can have a role in some children, but this, like other forms of treatment, is often ineffective. Children with conduct disorder tend to sabotage most forms of treatment.

While some children with conduct disorder will end up in prison, others do undergo a miraculous maturation in their late teens or early twenties and do not get into any further trouble. Many an adult who is now a good citizen had a very stormy childhood.

Summary points

- Approximately one quarter of children with ADD experience significant difficulties conforming to the ordinary rules and regulations that are appropriate for their age.
- Children with ADD who have non-compliant behaviour have parents who are no less competent than other parents. They are usually at their wit's end to know what to do with their extremely difficult children.
- A common aspect of such children's behaviour is its variability.
- Oppositional behaviour is milder and more common. Features include:
  active defiance
  argumentativeness
  temper outbursts
  annoying and provocative behaviour
  touchiness
  projection of blame

     resentfulness
     spitefulness and vindictiveness
     swearing

- Conduct disorder is more severe. Features include:
     stealing
     running away
     repeated lying
     setting fires
     truanting
     breaking in
     destruction of property
     physical cruelty to animals
     forced sexual activity
     using weapons
     initiating fights
     physical cruelty to people

- Early treatment of oppositional disorder makes the later development of conduct disorder less likely.
- Medication and counselling for the parents and child are the mainstays of treatment. Special educational units and residential units may be appropriate.
- Some children with conduct disorder do eventually settle down.

six

Social clumsiness

Children with ADD may experience social difficulties because of features of their condition, such as over-activity, impulsivity, and low self-esteem. In addition, many children with ADD have a limitation in the way in which their brain is able to understand and respond to social conventions. This is called a social cognition deficit.

Social cognition—a function of the brain

Much of what children learn about socially appropriate behaviour is not actually taught to them; they simply pick it up as they go along. For them to do this, certain parts of the brain need to develop to an appropriate maturity for the child's age. The child with ADD seems to have an immaturity in the part of the brain responsible for social cognition and so is less able to learn socially appropriate behaviour, even when taught.

Such a child experiences difficulty in behaving in a way that is socially appropriate for his age.

The people who are most likely to notice are the child's contemporaries, and as a result, he is often rejected by his peers. With his peers, such a child often sticks out as clearly different. Some are victimised and bullied. They often have a high profile because of their inappropriate behaviour. It is common for such children to be known by everyone in the school, but to have no friends.

Lack of friendship may make the child behave in an even more inappropriate way in order to gain attention. This is often the reason why such children will play the part of the class clown' or engage in provocative or eccentric behaviour.

Specific social competence deficits

'Social cognition deficit' describes deficits in a number of areas of social incompetence. A child with ADD may have one or more specific deficits. These include:

'Social blindness'

A 'socially blind' child has difficulty in reading a social situation so that behaviour can be adapted accordingly.

Children with this difficulty do not pick up the same social cues as other children of the same age. For example, they are likely to rush in to a social group and start talking when it is clear that the group should be approached in a quiet manner, and that they should watch, wait, and listen first.

Egocentricity

It is a characteristic of young children that they tend to be very self-centred. Children with ADD who have a social cognition defect will often behave in an egocentric way that is immature for their age. This will show itself in the fact that they will be 'bossy' with their peers. They want to dictate which games are played and insist on making, and often changing, the rules. They lack the degree of give-and-take that is appropriate for a child of their age.

Lack of appropriate inhibition

As normal children get older, they become more self-conscious and acutely aware of the need to behave in an appropriate manner for their age. Children with ADD may not develop such awareness and remain uninhibited. They may undress in public without the embarrassment that their peers would experience. They may be over-friendly to strangers. They may kiss classmates at an age when this is no longer appropriate. They may touch peers in a way that is not appropriate. None of these behaviours is carried out with any malice, but they evoke strong negative reactions. Some children with ADD make unusual sounds in public, such as imitating animal noises, in order to attract attention. This may irritate their peers.

Insatiability

This behaviour describes the tendency of children with ADD to behave in a certain manner without knowing when to stop. Such a child will be clearly differentiated from his peers who do know when 'enough is enough'.

Insensitivity to style and convention

Children with ADD are often not aware of those things that are considered essential for acceptance by their peer group. They may not notice appropriate dress or speech. They will then appear to be eccentric.

Children of a particular age generally use certain slang words and specific ways of expressing themselves that constitute 'child speak'. Children with ADD may have difficulty learning age-appropriate 'child-speak' and may speak, instead, in a way that sets them apart from other children of their age. They may not be as quick as other children in adapting to changes in style, so that they are still wearing last year's fashion when their peers have discarded it.

Lack of responsiveness

Many children with ADD are incapable of being receptive to other children's social initiatives. This is partly due to their egocentricity which makes them unable to subjugate their own desires in order to take the desires of others into account.

Over-talkativeness

Because of their impulsivity and social immaturity, many children with ADD have great difficulty being quiet. When they are anxious in a social group they become particularly talkative. Such garrulousness is quickly picked up by other children as being abnormal. It also means that the child is often very self-disclosing, talking about her own feelings and vulnerabilities, and this may encourage other children to bully and victimise her when they sense her weakness.

Poor metalinguistic skills

A particularly important area of development in children of school age is in the area of metalinguistic skills. This is the ability to analyse and reflect on language itself. Children with difficulties in this area will not be as competent as their peers in understanding metaphors, idioms, riddles, puns, jokes, and many other linguistic devices and nuances. Children with difficulties in this area will not be able to keep up with their more sophisticated peers. They will not understand jokes and may respond very literally to the things that their contemporaries say.

Difficulties reading facial expression

Children with ADD often have great difficulty reading facial expressions and may be oblivious to whether someone is angry or upset with them. They may therefore not modify their behaviour according to another person's response.

Aggressive tendencies

As children get older, they are more likely to resolve conflicts peacefully. Children with ADD, particularly those with oppositional disorder, tend to resort to verbal or physical violence when frustrated. They lack the normal aptitude for settling a disagreement amicably. This makes them unpopular.

Lack of judgement

Children with ADD may get themselves into all kinds of problems because of a lack of judgement. Often they will fight with children who are clearly larger and stronger than they. They may try to establish friendships with children who actually dislike them and whom they should leave alone; or they will persist in annoying another child to the point where they will receive a negative response from the whole group.

Poor understanding of group dynamics

Many children with ADD will manage well playing with one child at home. However, in the playground, where children often group together, they will have great difficulty. This may be because of difficulties with understanding group dynamics. Relating to other children as part of a group requires a subtle understanding of human relationships which is extremely difficult for a child with this kind of social cognitive deficit.

Pacing difficulties

Many children with ADD have great difficulties knowing when to do or say things, and are often too quick in their timing and staging of social discourse and activities.

Misinterpreting feedback

Children with ADD may misunderstand the cues that they are receiving from their peers. They may be insensitive to whether they are receiving negative or positive social feedback when relating to other children.

Tactlessness

Children with ADD are often very tactless. Without intending any harm they will blurt out inappropriate or hurtful statements. They are unable to understand that things should not be said in certain situations. Because of their difficulties in predicting outcomes, they are often very surprised by the negative reaction that their behaviour evokes. Sometimes they do not even notice other people's disapproval or hurt.

Poor social prediction

Children with ADD have great difficulties predicting the consequences of their actions. They typically have little or no insight into how differently they are perceived. Unfortunately, this makes it very difficult for them to learn the skills that are required to mix with other children.

Poor social memory

The lack of the ability to recall prior social experience makes it difficult for children with ADD to benefit from past experience.

Lack of awareness of image

Children with ADD will often not be able to present themselves to peers in a socially acceptable way because they are unable to see themselves as their peers view them.

Poor behaviour modification strategies

It is important for children to be able to understand and reinforce the feelings of their friends. Children with ADD often have difficulty with this because they are not in tune with their peers' feelings and lack the strategies for reinforcing responses.

Lack of correction strategies

To make things more difficult, children with ADD often have poor recuperative strategies to compensate for their social errors. Any child may make an error in social interaction, but most will then be able to compensate for this. Children with ADD have difficulties in this area and may, in an attempt to correct things, further compound their difficulties.

Management

Children with a social cognitive defect have a part of their brain that is immature relative to their peers. They would like to be liked and socially successful, but they do not yet have the ability to learn the necessary techniques.

It is all too easy to believe that helping a child with a social cognitive defect is simply a matter of teaching new strategies. It has to be realised that in many children with ADD one is dealing with a brain that is not yet ready to learn these strategies.

No amount of social skills training will help a child to behave in a socially appropriate way if he is not yet ready to understand and, more importantly, apply such skills. It is characteristic of children with this sort of difficulty that they may be able to behave in an appropriate way in a social skills group, but then have difficulty applying such behaviour in their day-to-day interactions.

Wherever possible, parents should try to help the child by modifying the environment in which she finds herself. Occasionally a change of school may be helpful; however, because the problems lie with the child, difficulties with social relationships may reappear in the new setting.

Parents may need to take an active role in arranging for another child to play with their child after school. Parents can also play a role by tactfully pointing out ways in which the child could win friends. It may be helpful to rehearse certain situations with your child so that he learns how to act in them. This should be done so that it is an enjoyable experience.

It is important to try to identify which particular aspects of social interaction are causing difficulties. For example, a child with difficulties understanding dress styles and with a poor awareness of his image may need the parent to keep an eye on appropriate fashions and to ensure that he is dressed in a way that blends in with his peers.

Some health centres and adolescent units run social skills training groups where children of all ages learn to better understand the social consequences of their actions. They can also acquire techniques for interpreting social cues and for being accepted by their peers.

Cognitive training may also be helpful. In this situation, the child is given one-to-one counselling by a professional trained in social skills development. The child can be taught techniques, such as to stop and think before acting. He is taught to first stop, then to focus and look at the possible ways he may act, and then, thirdly, to act according to a plan. The child is taught, lastly, to evaluate what has happened. Children who are well motivated may respond to this sort of help.

Medication can be extremely helpful to a child with a social cognition defect and may be used alone or in conjunction with other treatment. The medicines used for ADD will often improve behaviours that impair social relationships, such as disinhibition, impulsivity, garrulousness, and aggressive tendencies. Children with ADD are rated more positively by their peers when they are on medication.

Summary points

- Many children with ADD have a limitation in the way in which their brain is able to understand and respond to social conventions. This is called a social cognition deficit.
- Such children experience difficulty behaving in a way that is socially appropriate for their age. As a result, they are often rejected by their peers.
- Unfortunately, children with social cognition defects often become loners. Some are victimised and bullied by their peers.
- 'Social cognition deficit' describes deficits in a number of areas of social incompetence. A child with ADD may have one or more specific deficits. It is important to try to identify which particular aspects of social interaction the child is having difficulties with.
- Wherever possible, parents should try to help the child by modifying the environment in which she finds herself.
- Parents may need to take an active role in arranging for another child to play with their child after school.
- Some health centres and adolescent units run social skills training groups where children learn a better understanding of the social consequences of their actions. They can also acquire techniques for interpreting social cues and for being accepted by peers.

- Cognitive training may also be helpful. In this situation the child is given one-to-one counselling by a professional trained in social skills development.
- Medication can be an extremely effective way of helping a child with a social cognition defect and may be used alone, or in conjunction with other methods of treatment.

seven

Low self-esteem

It is hard to think of any attribute more crucial to success in life than high self-esteem. Whatever abilities a child may have, without a good self-image she is unlikely to succeed. If success does come to an individual with a low self-esteem, it is unlikely to be enjoyed.

Most children with ADD suffer from a low self-esteem. This may become apparent to the parents when the child makes negative comments such as 'I am dumb!' or 'I can't do this!' In some children, poor self-esteem may show itself by excessive moodiness, irritability, tearfulness, or withdrawal. In other children, problems with self-esteem may not be apparent. Difficult behaviours such as aggression, an excessive desire to control situations, distaste for being cuddled, and excessive quitting can all be attempts to maintain a fragile self-esteem. It is easy to misinterpret such behaviour as defiant or perverse. Unfortunately, if the origin of these behaviours is not recognised, attempts to correct them may further undermine the child's self-esteem.

Self appraisal—a function of the brain

We all know individuals who have been successful, but who have poor feelings of self-worth; and there are many people who have not been successful, or who have not had good experiences during their lives, who maintain a positive estimation of their own value.

It seems that there are important mechanisms in the brain that control the way in which children evaluate themselves and cope with things that go wrong in their day-to-day experience. Stella Chess and Alexander Thomas were the first to describe the noticeable differences in temperament that babies demonstrate almost immediately after birth. Studies of alteration of self-appraisal in adults who have undergone brain injuries, as well as after the effects of drugs that act on the brain, give further support to a biological, brain-based component to self-esteem.

While it is true that children with ADD often experience failure because of their condition, an important reason for their poor self-esteem may relate to immaturities in the self-appraisal mechanism of their brains. Not only is it difficult to manage as a child with ADD, but children with ADD are extremely hard on themselves.

The part of the brain that controls self-esteem is widely believed to be the limbic system which lies deep within the frontal part of the brain. The frontal parts of the brain receive highly processed and filtered sensory information from other parts of the brain. That information eventually reaches the limbic system, which regulates emotional responses and feelings. As explained in the following chapter, there is evidence that this part of the brain has not matured appropriately in children with ADD.

This would explain why many of the characteristics of self-appraisal in children with ADD are immature. For example, very young children tend to look for someone or something to blame for things that go wrong. A young child who hurts himself may become angry and aggressive, looking for someone else to blame for the accident. He therefore projects the 'locus of blame' onto his mother or siblings (or even an inanimate object). As children develop they become less likely to look for a locus of blame for things that go wrong. They can accept the fact that accidents occur, and shrug off difficulties with a reasonable amount of equanimity.

A child with ADD will often retain this tendency to look for a locus of blame beyond the age where it usually disappears. Misfortune may give rise to anger and aggression directed towards others who were not responsible for what happened.

Children with ADD will often project the locus of blame onto themselves and therefore appraise themselves harshly for things that go wrong. Conversely, if things go well they may not attribute this to their own ability. It becomes clear that they have not developed an appropriate feeling of autonomy or competence which is necessary for adequate feelings of self-worth. This can be seen in the way in which they respond to their achievements. A normal child who passes an examination will be able to feel good about his or her achievements. A child with ADD may say something like 'the questions were very easy', or 'the teacher gave me more marks because she knows I am dumb!'.

With an immature appraisal system, children with ADD can easily come to attribute negative intentions to other people when these intentions do not exist. They are therefore quick to feel threatened and discouraged. It is characteristic of many children with ADD that they always expect the worst and that they have difficulties in seeing good in others or themselves.

It is easy to see how children with ADD can become depressed. Depression is a form of anger directed at oneself, and children who project blame onto themselves, and feel that they are not capable or competent, can easily become sad and withdrawn.

Children with ADD are thus doubly at risk for problems with self-esteem. First, they have many difficulties in their everyday performance due to their problems with poor attention span, impulsivity, poor social cognition, and difficulties with learning. They therefore often experience failure and criticism. Second, they have problems with self-appraisal that lead them to quickly lose feelings of self-worth.

Control of the self-appraisal system in the brain

We still know little about how the self-appraisal system that controls self-esteem works. However, it seems certain that levels of neurotransmitters play an important role.

Neurotransmitters are chemicals produced at the end of nerves in the brain to send a message from one nerve cell to another. As will be discussed in the following chapter, low levels of certain neurotransmitters are believed to be the basic cause of ADD.

Although many people have difficulty understanding how chemicals in the brain can control self-esteem, most people have personal experience of temporarily 'adjusting' their self-appraisal mechanisms by changing the levels of neurotransmitter in the brain. They do this by drinking alcohol. Many people will have had the experience of feeling more capable after an alcoholic drink. For example, public speakers will sometimes have a drink of alcohol to 'steady their nerves' before speaking.

Alcohol works by altering neurotransmitter levels. (This is the way most drugs affect the brain.) The individual feels an improved feeling of self-worth and confidence while the alcohol is active. Alcohol often makes the speech worse, but nevertheless, the speaker *thinks* he is doing much better. This is a clear demonstration that actual performance need not be associated with self-esteem.

Drinking alcohol to 'steady the nerves' is to be avoided. However, it does demonstrate that self-esteem is at least partially controlled by neurotransmitters. The speaker who has fortified himself with alcohol becomes less competent and yet feels far more competent. Of course, once the alcohol wears off, confidence decreases and there might even be a rebound effect, whereby the individual feels that he has performed poorly.

Dysfunctional coping behaviours

Many unwanted behaviours that are seen in children with ADD are due to problems with self-esteem. It is essential that parents and teachers recognise this before trying to treat the behaviour. Often such behaviours cannot be eradicated without helping the child gain better feelings of self-worth, something that may take time.

It is very easy to become frustrated with these behaviours and criticise the child. However, this will only lower the child's feeling of self-worth further and entrench the behaviour, or force the child to substitute other unwanted behaviours.

All of these behaviours are attempts on the part of the child to deflect feelings of inadequacy and to prevent them from getting worse. In most cases the attempts are only partially successful, and treatment should aim to find successful ways of reducing the negative feelings.

Here are some examples of dysfunctional behaviours, together with some advice about managing them.

Quitting

Some children develop a habit of quitting as a way of coping with feelings of inadequacy. When frustrated, because they cannot win a game or accomplish a skill, they will quit. They often will offer an excuse, such as that the task or game was 'stupid' or 'boring'. In both school work and in games, they give up the moment they encounter difficulties and then refuse to continue.

It is no use entering into a discussion with the child about the importance of the activity, or insisting that it is not boring. The child's criticism of the activity is simply a smokescreen that she raises in order to protect herself from failure. Arguing about this is not going to resolve the issue. In fact, by arguing that the activity is important, you only increase her anxiety about failing.

It is important that you make certain that the tasks your child attempts are within his capabilities. If a task or game is difficult, try to find a substitute that is within his capabilities. Try to give him special jobs to do that require a small degree of persistence, and have a reward system for when he finishes these. In this way he will have the opportunity to learn that persistence does pay. Tell him stories about great people who did not give up when they were facing defeat. Children's libraries often have books that teach children particular virtues, like courage or persistence.

Most importantly, try to take the tension out of the situation. Make activities as much fun as possible. Join in where possible and show that you too make mistakes, but that you do not become upset.

Avoiding

Avoiding is similar to quitting, except the individual does not even start the activity. Children with ADD will often not want to join in activities, or to volunteer to take part, for fear of failing. Children with ADD often refuse to make arrangements to visit a friend, do not want to try for a part in a play, or will not put their hand up in class because of problems with poor self-esteem. Their feeling of self-worth is so low that they feel that they cannot afford to fail.

It is essential that such children should not be criticised. They need to be directed towards activities in which they can succeed and where they are not in the limelight.

Adverse responses to praise

Children with low self-esteem might behave in an adverse way when praised. Instead of enjoying praise, they may become angry or negative whenever praise is given. Because they feel so inadequate, any praise is misinterpreted and regarded as implied criticism. Praise often reminds them of how far they fall below their own expectations and what they believe to be the expectations of the person who is praising them. They interpret the praise as being patronising and containing implied criticism.

In such a situation, praise should be used sparingly and only when it is clear that the child feels satisfied with her performance. Praise the child's accomplishment rather than the child herself. Wherever possible, encourage the child to praise herself, but do not persevere if it is clear that she does not feel comfortable about doing this.

Tactile defensiveness

Children with ADD often do not like being touched or cuddled. This aversion to touch is known as 'tactile defensiveness'. Parents often become hurt at this, believing that the child does not feel affectionate towards them. The truth is that children with ADD often do not feel happy about being cuddled because of their low self-esteem. Often if a child does not feel good about himself, he will not enjoy being touched. This is because being cuddled makes him feel very vulnerable to rejection and because, strange as it may seem to the parent, the child does not feel loved or lovable.

Parents have to be patient with children who have tactile defensiveness. They have to strike a happy balance between not forcing themselves upon the child, and at the same time trying to make some physical contact that they hope will increase as the child becomes more confident. Knowing exactly what to do does require an ability to 'read' the child's feelings.

Parents naturally want to cuddle and comfort an upset child. However, children with ADD who have low self-esteem may be best left alone when they are upset, and may feel happiest sitting on their own or retreating to their room. The time to touch the child may be when the child is feeling happier and more confident. Touch should be very limited initially, increasing gradually as the child is desensitised. Many children with ADD benefit from having soft toys which they can cuddle without fear of rejection.

Cheating

Some children learn to cope with failure by cheating. This may occur at school, when work is copied, or at home. The child feels so certain that she cannot win a game or pass a test that she alters rules and copies answers.

You should make certain that your child is not being set tasks that are beyond her capabilities. You should also make certain that she is not receiving criticism for her failure. The child should be praised for her effort, even if her work is incorrect.

If teachers spot that a child is cheating, they should only mark the portion of the work that they feel the child has done herself and ignore the rest. In this way she learns that she is rewarded only for her own efforts.

It is best if you do not let your child get away with significant lying or cheating. Whenever she is caught at it, ask her if she understands what she is doing. Explain that you admire her efforts whether she succeeds or fails, but that cheating spoils games and work. Talk to her about this, mentioning that you understand why she wants to cheat, but explain how much better it is to be honest. Ensure that honesty is praised. In games, set an example of how to lose gracefully.

Lying

There are two forms of lying seen in children with ADD. Some children will lie in order to get what they want (offensive lying). This is to be discouraged and it is important for parents to ensure that children do not gain advantage by telling untruths.

A more common form of lying seen in children with ADD is when children lie to get out of trouble (defensive lying). This is a form of coping with low self-esteem. It is important not to put your child into a situation where he has to lie frequently. Parents should not ask their child if he is guilty when they suspect that he might have carried out some misdemeanour. By continually being put 'on the spot' in this way, the child is forced to lie in order to 'save face'. It is better if you only criticise your child when you know he has done something wrong.

In such a situation it is unnecessary for you to ask whether or not he was guilty. In those situations where you do not know if he has done something wrong, it would be better not to ask him difficult questions, whenever possible. Defensive lying often quickly resolves when parents cut down on the amount of cross-examining that they do.

Clowning

Children with low self-esteem will often play the part of the clown in order to gain attention and feel good about themselves. They will also feel that they can avoid activities in which they may fail by playing the part of the incompetent. Often children will inadvertently say something funny in class and then, when they realise the approbation that this brings, will continue to play this part. Other children are often only too willing to let the child with ADD make a fool of herself in this way. Unfortunately, clowning rarely wins true friends for the child and makes her susceptible to ridicule. She may then find it difficult for other children to take her seriously when she wants them to.

Clowning is usually seen in the classroom and it is important that teachers tackle this appropriately. Punishing the child who plays the part of the clown only decreases her self-worth and encourages further subversive clowning. Rather, the teacher should try to stop the other children from laughing at the child and thereby reinforcing her behaviour.

Regressive behaviour

Children often behave in an immature fashion as a way of coping with stress. Children with ADD who have self-esteem problems may behave in a babyish way because they are frightened of failing. By adopting a childish manner, they subconsciously hope to convey the impression that they are too young to be criticised for their failure. They tend to persist with this behaviour if it is successful.

A certain amount of regressive behaviour can be accepted, but if it is clear that the child is behaving in a babyish way too often, parents should make certain that mature behaviour is praised and regressive behaviour ignored and discouraged.

School avoidance

Children with ADD may avoid going to school. This may take a number of forms. The child may flatly refuse to leave home, he may frequently complain that he is ill, he may pretend that he is going off to school but never arrive, or he may leave school during the course of the day by absconding or saying he is ill.

Those who complain of being ill may be feigning illness, or they may be so anxious about going to school that they actually experience stress-related symptoms, such as abdominal pain and headaches.

This sort of school avoidance is usually due to distress about academic or social difficulties. He may be frightened of failing, or being teased or ostracised. Sometimes a child tries to avoid particular lessons, for example mathematics in the case of a child with particular difficulties with arithmetic, or physical education in a clumsy child. Parents may see a pattern in the days the child misses.

A distinction should be drawn between this sort of school avoidance and the intense fear of school (school phobia) that is often associated with issues related to leaving home, rather than anxiety about school itself.

If your child is avoiding school, speak to him about it. You should also speak to his teacher to see if there are academic or social stresses that can be reduced.

It is important to prevent school avoidance becoming a regular pattern of behaviour. If you feel that your child is feigning illness, do not give him excessive attention. Give him bland food when he is at home and do not let him spend time watching the TV. Be matter of fact and encourage attendance at school, even if only for half the day. It is important to keep in touch with the school and have work sent home which he is expected to do. There should be a clear expectation that he will return to school at the earliest possible opportunity.

If these simple measures do not work, it is best to involve your child's doctor or a psychologist. This is particularly important if your child is refusing to leave his room or if he is very withdrawn.

Homework avoidance

Homework avoidance often leads to a great deal of conflict between parents and children with ADD. If your child is not completing her homework, you should first check whether it is too difficult, or too much, for her. If so, speak to her teacher about this.

If the level and amount of homework is appropriate, but your child is still having difficulties, you may need to look at how she goes about the work. Do not be tempted to do the work for her, but help her learn to organise herself efficiently. You will need to look at when she does the homework, where she does it, and how she arranges the time to do it.

It is usually best if there is a specified homework time. For some children with ADD, this may need to follow a chance to burn off energy in active play. For other children, it may be better to leave the play as a reward for after the homework is completed. Whichever time is chosen, there should be some specified reward for when the work is completed. The child needs as quiet an environment as possible. Many children work best if there is a parent nearby, even though he or she may not need to take an active part in helping the child. For such children, the parent's presence has a settling effect. Homework should not go on for too long. If there is a lot of work to cover, or if your child is slow, it may need to be broken up into a couple of sessions.

It is important that you teach your child how to manage her time effectively. She needs to know how to arrange work according to priorities, and how to work systematically. Teach her not to expect you to do all the work for her, but to think of you as a resource that she can call upon when she needs advice.

Children may need particular help if a project needs to be completed over a long period. Help your child to break this into stages and to create a timetable for completing each stage. Without this help, things will often be left to the last minute and the child then feels overwhelmed.

TV 'addiction'

Parents of children with ADD often complain that their child spends a lot of time watching TV. Difficulties with academic work, as well as with social relationships, mean that TV is a common diversion for this group of children.

Limiting the amount of TV is only part of the answer. It is important to find rewarding substitute activities. You may be able to find after-school activities for your child, based on his interests. Keep an eye on local newspapers and talk to other parents to find out about suitable activities for children. You may also obtain information from local sports and recreation centres. If your child is having difficulties making friends, he may benefit from attending a social skills group. You need to check with your local health centre whether one is being run in your area.

Aggression

Aggressive behaviour is a common cover for low self-esteem. A child who feels that he has failed may vent his anger on others. A child who does not feel good about himself may derive satisfaction by exerting power over others. Such a child may get into fights, bully other children, or engage in arguments and make critical remarks about siblings and others.

Listen carefully to what your child says when he insults others; he is probably echoing the criticisms that hurt him most. If this is the case, you need to check on why he feels that he is being criticised in this way, and take steps to stop it. Check whether he is being victimised at school; he may be part of a pecking order and simply acting out the aggression he is experiencing.

Determine whether he is behaving aggressively only in certain situations and see if you can identify what provokes the behaviour. Often outbursts occur at times when your child feels a failure, or threat of failure. It may be possible to avoid such situations, or to change things so that your child does not feel inadequate.

For some children, it may be necessary to arrange a reward system for not losing their temper. You should also teach your child strategies for coping with his aggressive feelings. He may go for a walk, jump on a trampoline, or listen to music. Sometimes a child will benefit from a punch bag, or even a pillow on which he can vent his anger. Encourage him to express to you the way he feels and accept these feelings with sympathy.

If aggressive outbursts remain a problem despite these measures, it is a good idea to seek help from your child's doctor or psychologist. If the habit of resorting to aggressive outbursts becomes ingrained, it may be difficult to eradicate later and may cause much trouble in adulthood.

Controlling behaviour

Many children with low self-esteem feel that they have so little control over their own lives that they feel quite helpless. Some children respond by trying to command and dominate others. They tell people what to do, defy adults, and generally seek to dominate and control situations.

The best way to manage such behaviour is to give the child some areas where he does have control, for example choosing his clothes, helping to select items at the supermarket, and deciding how to spend his pocket money (within reason!). Allocate some pleasant task that becomes his responsibility and reward him for doing it. Explain that certain tasks are his domain but others are not.

When giving instructions, do this in the form of choices whenever possible: 'Do you want to tidy up your room while I do the lounge?', or 'Will you do the lounge while I do your room?'. This is less likely to make him feel that he is losing autonomy.

Passive aggression

Some children with ADD develop behaviour that is passively aggressive. There is no overt aggression, but the child subverts attempts to control her. For example, she will promise to meet certain responsibilities, but then 'forgets' to do so. She may sabotage attempts by parents to achieve goals by failing to turn up to planned activities when required. Such children avoid confrontation, but make it extremely difficult for parents to control them.

Management of passive aggressive behaviour combines techniques used for aggressive behaviour and for controlling behaviour. Children with passive aggressive behaviour should be given more control over their lives and allowed to express their anger verbally. Sometimes such children need individual counselling so that they can express their suppressed feelings of anger.

Denial

Another behaviour that is commonly seen in children with low self-esteem is a tendency to deny difficulties. In this way they can deal with the feelings of hurt that may result if they were to acknowledge their limitations and vulnerability. When asked about their concerns they will simply state that they do not care about things or that things are going well. Once more, counselling may be needed to help such children talk about their difficulties.

Rationalisation

As children with ADD get older they may start offering many excuses for their difficulties and failures. For example, a child caught cheating might argue that he was disadvantaged in some way in the examination and that therefore it was appropriate that he compensate for this by looking at someone else's work. After failing a test he may start criticising specific short-comings in the test as a way of maintaining his self-esteem.

With children who tend to rationalise, it is important not to become involved in arguments that attack their defences. Rather, it is important to recognise the origin of the child's rationalisation—the need to maintain self-esteem—and to find ways of bolstering the child's feelings. Sometimes all that is necessary is to listen to the child and acknowledge the feelings of frustration that he is experiencing.

Impulsivity

Impulsivity is a primary characteristic of ADD, but might also be seen as a response to difficulties with self-esteem. Children may cope with their difficulties by sudden impulsive acts in an attempt to 'just get it over with'.

The importance of self-esteem maintenance mechanisms

The behaviours discussed above are strategies that all children use at some time to maintain their self-esteem. Children with ADD are different in that they are more likely to use these mechanisms in a counter-productive way. They are not thought out by the children, but are strategies they come across by accident and then recruit as part of their protective shield. In all cases they are attempts by the child to maintain his or her feeling of self-worth.

The primary aim of any treatment should be to maintain the child's feeling of self-esteem. One can, therefore, not simply remove these defence mechanisms without putting something else in their place.

Summary points

- Many children with ADD suffer from low self-esteem.
- Children with ADD have many difficulties in their every-day performance due to their problems with poor atten-

tion span, impulsivity, poor social cognition, and difficulties with learning. In addition, they have problems with self-appraisal that lead them to lose feelings of self-worth.
- Many unwanted behaviours that are seen in children with ADD are due to problems with self-esteem.
- Behaviours caused by poor self-esteem include:
  quitting
  avoiding
  adverse response to praise
  tactile defensiveness
  cheating
  lying
  clowning
  regressive behaviour
  school avoidance
  homework avoidance
  'TV addiction'
  aggression
  controlling behaviour
  passive aggression
  denial
  rationalisation
  impulsivity
- The primary aim of any treatment of these behaviours should be to maintain the child's feeling of self-esteem. Ways should be found to help the child find more useful mechanisms to take the place of any that are undesirable.

The cause of ADD

eight

An immaturity of brain development

There is a tendency to attribute all difficulties that children have in learning or behaviour to 'bad parenting', or to some 'attitudinal' problem on the part of the child.

These ways of explaining children's difficulties arise from a number of traditions. First, people have for generations used terms such as 'naughty', 'lazy', and 'spoilt' without thinking carefully about the origins of children's behavioural and learning difficulties. Such phrases are handed down from parent to child as folk psychology.

Second, the writings of Sigmund Freud, which have greatly influenced the thinking of many lay people and professionals, largely interpret children's behaviour in the light of their early experiences.

Third, this century has seen many psychologists trained by behaviourists, who emphasise that behaviour is learned. Behaviourism is based on research involving laboratory animals and the work of people such as Pavlov and Skinner.

The belief that behaviour is determined by external factors has only recently been questioned. There is growing acceptance that children's brains develop at different rates, and that immature brains give rise to immaturities of behaviour that are not a consequence of the environment. Most important has been the realisation that, in order to help many children with learning and behavioural difficulties, we may need to treat the basic immaturity of the brain. It is now recognised that for such children treatment with counselling and behavioural training *alone* is often doomed to fail.

Not all skills are taught

Many of the skills that children develop are not taught to them. The classic example is walking. Children do not receive 'walking lessons'.

Some time between nine to eighteen months of age, a child's brain develops spontaneously to the point where walking becomes possible, and only then can the child walk. A child cannot walk before the nervous system has reached the necessary degree of maturity, and no amount of encouragement or training will make a child succeed prior to this time.

The *fundamental* difficulties experienced by children with ADD, such as poor attention and poor short-term memory, involve skills that, like walking, require development of the brain. These fundamental difficulties also influence the child's attainments in other areas, such as mathematics and spelling, that do require teaching.

As normal children grow older, they spontaneously develop competence in those areas where children with ADD experience difficulty. For example, normal children become more competent in concentrating as they grow older. When younger, they can only concentrate for short periods of time; and then only when they are very interested in something. As they develop, the concentration mechanism in their brains becomes more competent. They can concentrate on things that are not inherently so interesting, they can concentrate even when there are some distractions, and they can concentrate for the sake of some intangible goal to be realised far off in the future. Similarly, as children grow older, they can sit still for longer periods of time, they become more persistent with tasks, they become less impulsive, they become more flexible in their relationships, they can defer gratification, they can cope better with frustration. In all these ways they become more mature because of changes that occur in their brains.

The particular skills children with ADD experience difficulty with are known as the *executive functions* of the brain. These are listed in Table 2. As children grow older, these functions develop and performance in each of these areas becomes more consistent and reliable. Executive functions seem to be carried out in the frontal part of the brain, the part behind the forehead.

Table 2   Executive functions of the brain

Sustained attention	Self-appraisal
Reflection	Social cognition
Temporary immobilisation	Compliance
Self-organisation	Short-term memory
Self-regulation	Coordination of movement

Different rates of development

Just as some children are late to get their first teeth, or to develop the changes of puberty, it seems that some children are late to increase the competence of the frontal part of their brains. Delay in such an important part of the brain, in a school-aged child, has very important consequences for learning and behaviour. It means that a normal, intelligent child may differ markedly from his peers in the consistency with which he can learn and behave.

The best way to understand a child with ADD is to think of him as being like a younger child in those areas in which he is experiencing difficulty. The basic difficulty for the child with ADD is that, when he needs to concentrate, to sit still, to understand social situations, he is doing so with brain mechanisms that are immature and inefficient. It is not that he cannot do these things at all. Rather, the problem is that, like a younger child, he cannot do these things as *consistently* as other children of the same age. It is this performance inconsistency, the 'Jekyll and Hyde' nature of children with ADD, that is so confusing.

To understand this inconsistency, it is necessary to appreciate that a developmental skill is not attained suddenly. Rather, the child slowly becomes more and more consistent in his ability to perform a particular skill over time. The best way to understand this is to view skill acquisition as going through three stages.

The three stages of skill acquisition

Figure 1 shows a representation of the three stages of skill acquisition for walking.

Initially, the infant cannot walk at all—the stage of *incompetence* for this skill.

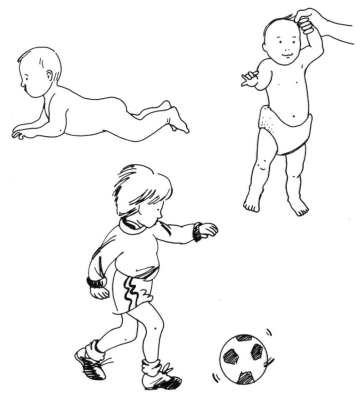

Figure 1   The three stages of skill acquisition for walking: incompetence (above left), inconsistency (above right), and competence (below).

Next, he reaches a stage when he can take a few steps if supported, but quickly loses his balance. At this stage the child cannot walk quickly and becomes unstable if the terrain is not flat. This is the stage of *inconsistency* for this skill.

Eventually, his ability becomes more and more consistent and he becomes a competent walker. Now he does not tire easily, he can walk for long periods, and he remains stable on all kinds of terrain. He has reached the stage of *competence* for the skill.

For many developmental skills, the child with ADD is stuck in the second stage of skill acquisition (inconsistency) when his contemporaries have already attained the stage of competence. Because he is delayed in his development, he remains in this stage for longer than usual. For example, when his peers can concentrate on tedious tasks for long periods (stage of competence for attention), he is still easily distracted unless the task is interesting (stage of inconsistency).

The performance inconsistency that children with ADD experience will be better understood if this three-stage model is kept in mind.

Normal brain development—ages and stages

As children grow their bodies change. We are all familiar with the physical changes that occur in children's bodies at puberty. These changes are controlled by a 'genetic clock' that switches on certain genes at critical ages.

The brain, too, is under the control of a genetic clock that allows certain parts of the brain to become more influential as the child grows older. These are parts of the brain involved in executive functions such as concentration, reflection (stopping to think so as not to act impulsively), and social cognition ('reading' social situations in order to act appropriately). These vital executive functions of the brain play a role in controlling the performance of the individual. The Swiss psychologist Jean Piaget detailed the way many of these functions change with age.

How does the brain develop?

What changes in the brain so that executive functions become more mature? This is not a question that can be answered with certainty, yet we now have so many pieces of this puzzle that it is not difficult to see the complete picture. To explain it will require some simplification.

The brain is composed of a network of approximately 100 billion nerve cells. Messages flow along nerves in a way that is comparable to electricity travelling through a wire. Adjoining nerve cells communicate by releasing neurotransmitter molecules which traverse the gaps (synapses) between them. Figure 2 shows the end of a nerve cell and the neurotransmitter it produces to transmit its message to the next nerve cell.

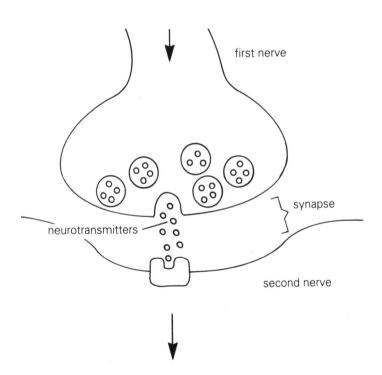

Figure 2   The synapse between two nerve cells.

The brain does not acquire any new brain cells after birth. For a part of the brain to start exerting a greater influence on behaviour, nerve cells already present in that part of the brain must become more powerful. This is believed to occur by the relevant brain cells increasing the amount of neurotransmitter that they produce. (It could also happen by the relevant brain cells producing extra branches, but their effect would still take place through a greater overall load of neurotransmitter.)

By increasing the amount of neurotransmitter it produces, a nerve cell is able to play a greater role in brain function. It becomes more influential in the working of the brain.

As a child's brain develops, it is likely that more neurotransmitter is produced in the frontal part of the brain. As described earlier, this part of the brain is involved in controlling executive functions, such as attention, short-term memory, reflection, and social cognition. The stronger influence of this part of the brain allows the child to become more consistent in her ability to concentrate, more able to think before she acts, more tactful in her dealings with others, to name just a few results. All of these are functions with which children with

Table 3   Executive functions of the brain with the corresponding features of ADD

Executive Function	Feature of ADD
Sustained attention	Poor concentration
Reflection	Impulsivity
Temporary immobilisation	Overactivity
Self-organisation	Lack of planning
Self-regulation	Inflexibility
Self-appraisal	Poor self-esteem
Social cognition	Social clumsiness
Compliance	Defiant behaviour
Short-term memory	Forgetfulness
Coordination of movement	Clumsiness

ADD have difficulty. Table 3 matches up the executive functions of the brain with the corresponding features of ADD.

It is now widely believed that in ADD the levels of certain neurotransmitters in the frontal part of the brain do not increase adequately with age. This is known as the *neurotransmitter theory of ADD*. Two neurotransmitters are involved: *dopamine* and *norepinephrine*. (At one stage the neurotransmitter serotonin was also implicated, but its involvement seems to be less likely.)

Evidence for the neurotransmitter theory

Neurotransmitter levels in the living brain cannot be measured directly. Support for the neurotransmitter theory is, therefore, based on indirect information from a number of sources. When combined, these provide extremely strong evidence that ADD is due to a depletion of neurotransmitter in the frontal part of the brain. These sources include:

Neuropharmacology

The study of how drugs affect the nervous system has given us insights into how neurotransmitters work at nerve endings. All the medicines used in ADD act by altering neurotransmitter levels.

Cognitive neuroscience

The study of the structure and function of the simple brains of some animals has allowed us to understand the role of neurotransmitters in brain functions such as attention and memory.

Developmental neurobiology

The study of how the brain changes with age has shown that the detailed structure of the brain is continually modified by an interplay of environmental and genetic determinants.

Neuropathology

The study of the effect of different brain injuries and diseases on brain function has linked particular parts of the brain with specific executive functions. This has been supplemented by information obtained by stimulating specific parts of the brain with an electric probe. The subjects, who were conscious at the time, described the sensations elicited by the stimulation. Most of this work was carried out by Penfield and Roberts in the 1950s.

PET scanning

A type of scan that shows which part of the brain is active at any one time, PET scanning has shown that the frontal regions of the brains of individuals with ADD function inadequately when the subject is carrying out specific executive functions.

The most important PET studies carried out in people with ADD have been those by Hans Lou in Denmark (children) and Alan Zemetkin in the USA (adults). Lou showed that the abnormalities on the PET scans of children with ADD decreased when a medicine (Ritalin) used to treat ADD was given. Ritalin increases the levels of the neurotransmitter dopamine.

Neuro-electrophysiological studies

Sophisticated neuro-electrophysiological studies measuring the electrical activity of the brain are now commonly available and demonstrate that the brain function of individuals with ADD is immature and inefficient when carrying out certain attentional and learning tasks. These measures are now used in the diagnosis of ADD and are described in the next chapter.

As in the case of PET scans, abnormalities shown on neuro-electrophysiological tests are often reduced dramatically when medicine to increase neurotransmitter levels is administered.

Neuropsychology

Neuropsychology is a branch of psychology that allows careful measurement of specific skills. This has enabled difficulties in children with ADD to be detected and accurately measured so that they can be correlated with particular parts of the brain.

Animal models

Animals whose learning and behaviour closely parallels the disorder have been studied. 6-OHDA is a chemical that selectively destroys dopamine production, and insertion of 6-OHDA into the brains of rat pups, produces a condition identical to ADD. The rats respond to the same medicines used in humans with ADD and usually grow out of their condition, in the same way that humans do.

Depletion of neurotransmitters

The production of neurotransmitters consists of a number of steps.

The neurotransmitter must be manufactured in the cell from its basic components (*synthesis*). It must then be stored in small containers in the cell, called the storage vesicles. When a nerve impulse traverses the cell, the neurotransmitter must be *released* from the nerve end. The neurotransmitter then exerts its action by attaching (*binding*) itself to a receptor on the next cell, causing it to fire (send a signal in turn).

Other factors also come into play. The amount of neurotransmitter present in the synapse will not only depend on the amount released by the nerve ending, but also on how quickly it is *broken down*, and thus inactivated, by enzymes present in the synapse.

Some of the released neurotransmitter is reabsorbed by the cell that manufactured it, and can be reused (*re-uptake*).

There are also some feedback mechanisms that allow the cell to gauge whether there is sufficient neurotransmitter in the synapse or not. This is determined by *autoreceptors* on the nerve ending that produce the neurotransmitter. Any excess neurotransmitter in the synapse binds to the autoreceptors. If the autoreceptors are vacant, more neurotransmitter is released.

The suggested immaturities in the neurotransmitter mechanism in ADD result in there being smaller amounts of dopamine and/or norepinephrine in the synapse than are needed to transmit a nerve signal. This may be due to insufficient synthesis, inadequate release, excessive breakdown, or faulty feedback mechanisms. Some children probably have a combination of problems.

Any of these difficulties ultimately results in the same effect—inadequate amounts of the neurotransmitter. This effectively causes a 'blockage' in the nervous system. When a message is required in the part of the brain needed for an executive function, such as controlling impulsivity, concentrating, or for short-term memory, the message is not able to travel from one nerve cell to another.

The genetics of ADD

Each child inherits from his or her parents genes that control synthesis of neurotransmitters. It is quite in keeping with the neurotransmitter theory therefore that heredity is the most important factor in the causation of ADD.

ADD may be inherited from the child's father or mother. Recent research shows that in approximately 25% of cases it is the father, in about 20% the mother.

If one child in the family has ADD, there is more than a 35% chance of a brother or sister having the condition as well.

ADD does not always 'breed true'. That is, ADD may occur in different forms in different family members. Similarly, not all affected members of a family are necessarily helped by the same medicine.

Summary points

- Children's brains develop at different rates. This may give rise to immaturities of behaviour that are not a consequence of the child's environment.
- The fundamental difficulties experienced by children with ADD, such as poor attention and defective short-term memory, involve skills that, like walking, require development of the brain.

- The particular skills that children with ADD have difficulty with are known as the *executive functions* of the brain. As children grow older, these functions develop, and performance in each of these areas becomes more consistent and reliable.
- The brain is believed to be under the control of a *genetic clock* that allows certain parts of the brain to become more influential as the child grows older.
- Evidence from many sources points to neurotransmitter depletion in the frontal part of the brain as the cause of ADD.
- Heredity is the most important factor in the causation of ADD.

How ADD is diagnosed

nine

Diagnosis and assessment

- The first step in the proper treatment of ADD is making the diagnosis. Only when it is known that a child has ADD and that all other possible causes of the problems have been excluded, can a proper treatment programme be devised.

  The best person to make the diagnosis is a specialist paediatrician with an interest and expertise in the area of developmental and learning difficulties in children. Such 'developmental paediatricians' work in close liaison with educational psychologists, who play a vital role in the process by which ADD is diagnosed.

- Diagnosis involves a number of steps. First, a careful history must be taken to collect information about how the child learns and behaves at home and at school. Often this will require that parents and the teachers fill out a standard questionnaire which has been designed to help make the diagnosis of ADD.

- Second, the paediatrician will carefully examine the child to ensure that there is no other condition interfering with his learning and or behaviour.

- Third, special (psychometric) tests will need to be performed to develop an understanding of the child's particular areas of difficulty.

- Fourth, neuro-electrophysiological testing provides an objective measure of brain function.

It is then the responsibility of the paediatrician to evaluate all this information and to come to a diagnosis which he or she should explain to the parents.

The history

The paediatrician will ask questions in order to ascertain the child's special problems. He or she will want to know how long the parents have been concerned about the child, what concerns them, and which treatments have already been tried.

He or she will want to look at school reports to find out how the child is progressing and how teachers have evaluated the child over the years.

School reports are often written in an overly positive way because the teacher knows that the child will be reading the report and does not want to discourage him. It is therefore useful to ask the teacher to write a special letter for the paediatrician outlining the teacher's concerns about the child.

In some cases the teacher could be given a special check-list designed for children with ADD in which he or she can tick off those symptoms that have been noted in the classroom.

Sometimes it is best if the teacher, with the parents' permission, rings the doctor to give a first-hand description of the child's behaviour.

It is a good idea to obtain reports from other professionals who have seen the child in the past, and to show these to the paediatrician.

The paediatrician will also ask the parents about how their child behaves at home. It is best if both parents attend the assessment to enable both to give their views about the child. This will also allow both parents to hear the results and recommendations, and to have a say in any treatment plan which is developed.

The paediatrician will ask about the pregnancy and birth as well as about any health problems that the child has had. He or she will want to ensure that the child has adequate vision and hearing. It is a good idea to have both of these things checked before seeing the paediatrician. This should be done even if hearing and vision seem to be good in everyday situations, as minor difficulties are easily missed and may play a role in the child's learning problems. The family doctor will be able to arrange a referral to an ophthalmologist (a doctor specialising in eye disorders) and an audiologist (a technician trained to test hearing). If this cannot be organised before the consultation with the paediatrician, he or she may arrange for such testing to be done after the consultation.

The paediatrician will also enquire about any difficulties that may have been experienced by other family members. ADD, as well as other learning difficulties, may run in families and it is very useful in understanding the condition to know about other affected family members. It is a good idea for parents to ask their own parents about other family members before seeing the paediatrician.

The paediatrician may also give parents a questionnaire to fill in to obtain more detailed information about the child's behaviour. These questionnaires are used as a guide and have been administered to many thousands of parents in order to obtain an idea of what constitutes normal behaviour.

The examination

It is essential that the paediatrician carefully examines the child to ensure that he or she does not have a condition that interferes with learning. He or she will check the child's growth (height, weight, and head size). He or she will search for any unusual features in the child's body that suggest one of the rare genetic syndromes that are associated with learning difficulties.

The paediatrician will examine the nervous system with particular care looking for any abnormality ('hard' neurological signs). This is done by checking the child's balance and coordination, as well as muscular strength, muscular tone, and reflexes. He or she will also test the functioning of various nerves in the body.

Developmental paediatricians also look for 'soft' neurological signs, which are more subtle signs of immaturity in the way in which the brain processes sensations and controls movements. These signs do not have the same implications as hard neurological signs, but do indicate that the child is not yet functioning as maturely as other children of his age. Soft neurological signs are very common in children with ADD.

There are a number of conditions that the paediatrician needs to exclude before a diagnosis of ADD can be made. He or she needs to know that the child does not have a vision or hearing impairment which is causing the problem. Intellectual disability must be excluded. Physical disability, such as cerebral palsy, must also be excluded. Such conditions may be present in some children, but may not explain all the child's difficulties. They may act as an aggravating factor in a child whose primary problem is ADD. For example, a child may have mild intellectual disability, but may have problems with concentration and impulsivity that are excessive for his degree of intellectual disability. Such a child may have ADD as well as intellectual disability and may benefit from treatment of the ADD.

Psychometric testing

Careful evaluation of a child's particular areas of strength and weakness is essential in order to make the correct diagnosis, as well as to plan appropriate strategies for helping the child. It is only by this sort of evaluation that children with certain conditions that mimic ADD, such as intellectual disability, can be identified.

Once the child's particular areas of strength and weakness are established, an individualised treatment programme can be planned. For example, a child with ADD who has reading problems will need a different sort of help from the child with ADD who is a proficient reader.

The evaluation of a child's particular areas of strength and weakness requires individualised testing by an experienced educational psychologist using a battery of standardised 'psychometric' tests. The tests that are generally used have been administered to many hundreds of children to obtain standards for different ages. They have been carefully devised to compare an individual child's skills to those of his or her contemporaries. In this way one can determine whether a child is advanced, delayed, or age appropriate in different areas of development.

Tasks are presented in a specific order with the easier ones first. They then become progressively more advanced to establish at what level they become too difficult for the child. Every child who does the test will be presented with tasks that are easy, as well as tasks that are too difficult for him. This is necessary in order to find out the exact level at which he is functioning.

During the course of the test, a picture of the child's developmental progress can be formed, both for specific areas of development and for development as a whole. Sometimes a great deal of information can be gained from the way in which the child tackles tasks, even if he is unable to succeed. For example, the psychologist will observe his ability to persist with tasks, to attend for long periods, and to sit still.

The psychologist will choose tests that are most useful for the particular child. There are now many tests available and the psychologist will usually select a number of these. Children with suspected ADD should be given a test of intelligence, tests of academic achievement, and certain other tests of special ability.

Tests of intelligence

Although intelligence tests have come in for criticism over the past few years, they still form an essential part of establishing a child's abilities and needs. They must be performed by an experienced educational psychologist, and interpreted with care. The results of the tests should be regarded as only part of the child's assessment and need to be interpreted in the light of reports of his or her abilities at other times and the results of any previous tests.

Intelligence tests assess general intelligence. Many are very well suited to children with learning difficulties because they do not involve any reading or writing. They can, therefore, test intelligence irrespective of academic achievement. Intelligence tests not only establish the child's level of general intelligence, but also give valuable information about individual components of intelligence, such as short-term memory and sequential processing.

The different tasks in the most widely used intelligence tests are usually grouped into a number of 'sub-tests'; the score of each sub-test reflects a particular area of intelligence. The sub-tests for one of the commonest intelligence tests for school age children, the Wechsler Intelligence Scale for Children—third version (WISC–III) are grouped together to give a *verbal score*, which is a measure of the child's ability in language-related tasks, and a *performance score*, which is related to visual and manual tasks. A comparison of these scores will show if a child is having particular difficulties in one of these areas.

Another useful score which can be obtained from the WISC–III is known as the *freedom from distractability index* which refers to the child's performance on those parts of the test that require persistence with tedious tasks. Many, but not all, children with ADD score poorly in this area.

In interpreting these various components of intelligence tests, it is important to keep in mind the child's overall level of skill. For example, a highly intelligent child who is functioning in the 'superior' range may be regarded as having difficulties in concentration if his score in the *freedom from distractability index* is only in the 'average' range. On the other hand, such a score in the *freedom from distractability index* would be considered acceptable in a child whose overall intellectual function was also in the 'average' range.

Tests of academic achievement

These include tests of reading, spelling, and mathematics. It is essential that all children with ADD have these tests in addition to an intelligence test. It is not uncommon for a child who is thought to be functioning adequately at school to be found to have an unrecognised difficulty in one or more aspects of academic competence.

Academic achievement tests establish the level of a child's skills in a particular area of learning compared to her peers and also give important information about the nature of a child's difficulties in the area tested. The results will be given in terms of an age equivalency, i.e. the age at which the average child is able to function in the same way as the child who was tested. Some test results are expressed in 'percentiles', which indicate the percentage of children who would function less well at the same age. For example, a child with spelling competence on the 45th centile would be functioning better than 44% of children of the same age (and less well than 55% of children of the same age).

These tests compare children to others of the same age. Allowance may be necessary for children who started school at a later age than usual. Having been at school for a shorter period of time than most children of their age, it should be anticipated that their academic attainments will reflect this, rather than any lack of potential on the child's part.

Reading tests

Because the written word constitutes one of the most important ways in which children learn, reading is one of the most vital skills for children to acquire. The child with slow or inaccurate reading, and/or difficulties with reading comprehension, is at a great disadvantage. Reading difficulties are common in children with ADD.

There are a number of reading tests available to psychologists. Usually the child will be asked to read aloud from portions of text that have been graded according to difficulty. These texts have few, simple words in large print, often with illustrations. The child will progress to more and more difficult levels until it is clear to the tester that the child has reached her limit.

The tests usually determine the child's reading speed relative to other children of her age. The number of errors the child makes is also noted to establish reading accuracy, which is compared to age standards. After each portion of text is read, the tester may ask the child a number of standardised questions about what she has just read to determine the child's reading comprehension. This too can be compared to age standards.

Reading speed, accuracy, and comprehension can all be expressed in age levels. For example, a child of 9 years and 2 months may have a reading accuracy at a 6 year 3 month level, if she makes the same number of mistakes as the average 6 year 3 month old; and a reading comprehension age of 6 years 5 months, if she understands what she has read as well as an average 6 year 5 month old.

In addition to these scores, the tester is interested in the particular types of errors the child makes. He or she may also give the child some specific tests to try to establish the exact nature of the reading problem. For example, he or she may test the child's visual perception: the brain's ability to make sense of what is seen. He or she may compare the child's ability to read real and nonsense words to evaluate her phonological (sounding out) skills.

Many children with ADD will be found to have difficulties with reading speed, accuracy, and reading comprehension. In such children, it is important to distinguish those who have difficulties with reading comprehension *per se* and those whose reading comprehension simply reflects the fact that they are inaccurate readers. Some children may be able to understand something that is read fluently to them, but have difficulty extracting the meaning of something they read themselves. This does not indicate any difficulty with verbal comprehension, but simply difficulties with the process of reading itself. The remedial help for such a child would need to concentrate on reading accuracy. Reading comprehension would then improve. Other children may have difficulties understanding language and will need help in verbal comprehension. This requires the involvement of a speech therapist.

There are many children who find it embarrassing to read out aloud. For such children, a reading test that requires reading a passage to the psychologist may under-estimate their true reading accuracy and comprehension. It is impossible to measure reading accuracy without having the child read aloud, but it may be helpful to have the child read a passage silently to herself before asking questions that determine her reading comprehension. There are tests for measuring silent reading comprehension.

• Spelling tests

Spelling is another important area that should be assessed. There are several standardised spelling tests in general use. These differ in the way in which they test spelling. Some present the child with words that are part of his sight vocabulary, others present a wider range of words. Tests usually involve spelling from dictation. Some may also involve recognising whether a printed word is correctly spelt or not.

The psychologist will choose the test or tests that provide information about the child's spelling level, as well as about the nature of his difficulties. For example, a test that shows that a child has difficulties with spelling from dictation, but not with identifying words that are incorrectly spelt, may demonstrate particular problems with auditory discrimination (distinguishing sounds) or word memory.

The psychologist will also try to differentiate between different kinds of spelling errors, such as phonetic (words that look right but sound wrong), visual (words that sound right but look wrong), and sequential errors (for example 'brigde' for 'bridge').

• Arithmetic tests

The assessment of arithmetic skills becomes more difficult as children reach higher levels of proficiency in mathematics. For younger children, or children with significant difficulties in arithmetic, the psychologist may obtain sufficient information about the child's arithmetical ability from the *Arithmetic* sub-test of the WISC–III. This test does not require the child to write down the answers. The problems are timed and relate to various arithmetical skills.

Addition, subtraction, multiplication and division can all be tested. Some problems also require memorised number facts and subtle operations, such as seeing relevant relationships at a glance. The emphasis of the test is not on mathematical knowledge as such, but on mental computations and concentration.

The WISC–III will also give the psychologist information about other abilities that relate to arithmetical processes. In the *Digit span* sub-test, the child's ability to remember numbers for a short period is tested. This is a measure of working memory, an essential part of carrying out arithmetical operations in the brain. For example, in order to add 2 to 3, the 2 must be held in the working memory while 3 is added to it. Children with ADD often have low scores in the Digit span sub-tests. This partly relates to difficulties with working memory and partly to difficulties with auditory attention span.

In the *Comprehension* sub-test, verbal reasoning is involved. If, for example, a child has high comprehension but low arithmetic scores, this may suggest that reasoning ability is adequate in social situations, but not in situations involving numbers.

If the psychologist wants further information on arithmetical ability, there are a number of tests that specifically test mathematical skills and enable the results to be compared with those of children of the same age. They may also allow the psychologist to diagnose the precise difficulty that is interfering with the child's arithmetical performance. This will allow the remedial teacher to devise methods of providing specific help in the area of difficulty.

Tests of other special abilities

Children with suspected ADD should have careful assessment of their auditory and visual attention span, using standardised tests. There are specific tests for skills such as vigilance (ability to allocate attention to a new stimulus), task persistence, distractability, and short-term (working) memory.

These tests may be computerised. For example, in one commonly used test of vigilance, the child has to push a button whenever a particular number sequence (the stimulus) appears on the computer screen. The computer analyses the child's performance and compares it to standards for his age.

Such tests play an important part in helping the developmental paediatrician to make the diagnosis of ADD. They cannot be used in isolation, but form part of the information that is required to determine whether the child has ADD or not. They may also play an important role in determining the child's response to treatment and in reviewing the child's progress over time.

Many children with ADD have difficulties with handwriting. It is impossible to score a sample of writing in a precise way. Samples of writing are usually evaluated by an experienced tester. Three samples of writing are obtained: a passage of free composition on a particular topic, a piece of dictation, and a copy of some printed material. In the case of the free composition, the child is usually given a limited amount of time, such as five minutes. In the other two tests, he is timed to see how long he takes. In this way, the tester can see how quickly the child writes, as well as assess the legibility of the samples and study them to determine the nature of the child's difficulty. He or she will also observe the child's posture and method of holding the pen or pencil.

In addition to the writing test, the psychologist may do other tests, such as tests of drawing and visual perception.

Children with ADD often have difficulties with written expression. They find it very difficult to write about a topic. Children commonly say that the writing 'won't come'.

Children with difficulties with handwriting or with other fine motor skills, such as drawing, using scissors, or tying knots, should have standardised tests performed by an occupational therapist. Children with gross motor difficulty, in such activities as walking, running, jumping, hopping, or bicycle riding, may need to be referred by the developmental paediatrician to a physiotherapist for standardised testing.

Children with ADD often have difficulties with language. These may affect receptive language (understanding), expressive language (the ability to put words together) or speech (the clarity of the spoken word). A child with suspected language difficulties should be assessed by a speech therapist (sometimes called a speech pathologist). Such an assessment involves both informal observation and standardised tests to evaluate speech, expressive language, and receptive language. In addition to establishing the child's level of development in these areas, the speech therapist will determine the specific nature of his difficulties. No such testing should be performed until the child's hearing has also been properly tested.

Neuro-electrophysiological (neurometric) testing

Observations of how a child behaves or learns are extremely useful in the diagnosis of ADD. However, it can be difficult to know whether a child who performs poorly is doing so because of genuine difficulties or because they have poor motivation. It is therefore very useful to have ways of objectively assessing a child's brain to detect immaturities and inefficiencies of function.

The most suitable tests for general use are the neuro-electrophysiological tests. They do not require an injection, do not involve the use of any radiation, and cause no discomfort to the child. They are completely safe.

The usual test takes approximately one hour. A special fabric cap is placed on the child's head. The cap has wires connected to a sophisticated computer. The computer analyses the brainwaves produced by the brain while the child carries out three tasks: concentrating on a special pattern produced on a screen, counting intermittent tones produced through headphones, and sitting still with the eyes closed. The results of this testing gives rise to a scan of the brain known as a QEEG and a composite of brain wave patterns known as a cognitive event-related potential.

QEEG

Computerised quantitative analysis of EEG signals (QEEG) allows brain activity to be compared to that of a normal child of the same age, using stored data. This work was pioneered by Frank Duffy at Boston University and E. Roy John at New York University. Important contributions to our knowledge of the QEEG characteristics of ADD have been made by Christopher Mann and his associates from the University of Tennessee.

Children with ADD characteristically have immature activity in the frontal part of the brain. This can be shown on a picture known as a BrainMap that represents the numerical findings of the QEEG in a pictorial form.

A BrainMap of a normal child is compared to a characteristic BrainMap seen in ADD in Figure 3. In the child with ADD, the frontal part of the brain shows excess immature activity in the form of slow (theta) wave activity. It can be seen that this appearance is corrected by medication taken for ADD.

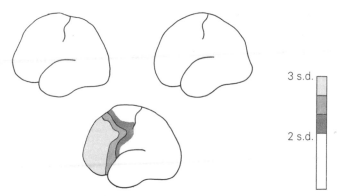

Figure 3 BrainMaps: Normal (above left), ADD before treatment (below), ADD after treatment (above right). The shaded area shows excess theta activity for age [s.d. = standard deviations].

Cognitive event-related potential

The second type of information obtained from neuro-electro-physiological testing relates to what is known as 'a cognitive event-related potential' (ERP).

A cognitive event-related potential measures changes in the electrical activity of the brain that occur when specific tasks are undertaken.

For example, when asked to listen for a sound, a child must allocate attention, and an event-related potential recorded when the child attends to the sound will contain elements that reflect the deployment of attentional capacity that takes place in the brain.

Rafael Klorman and his associates from the University of Rochester have confirmed the work of many researchers that demonstrate inefficient attentional allocation mechanisms in children with ADD. When children with ADD concentrate

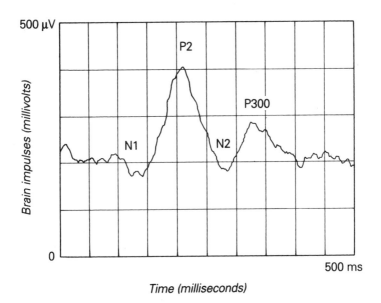

Figure 4　A normal cognitive event-related potential.

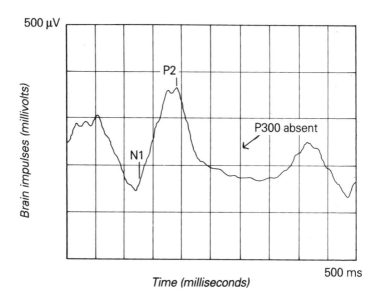

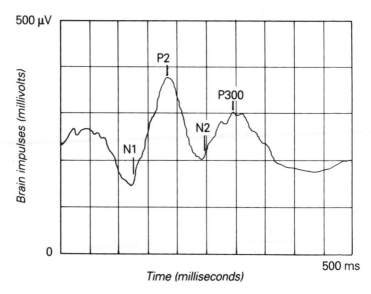

Figure 5 Cognitive event-related potential: ADD before treatment (above), ADD after treatment (below).

intently on a sound, they do not generate the strong waves on cognitive event-related potentials that normal children do. In children with ADD, certain waves on cognitive event-related potentials are smaller and occur later.

Figure 4 shows the cognitive event-related potential of a normal child who is having to count tones heard infrequently. A wave, known as the P300, indicates that the attentional mechanism is working efficiently.

Figure 5 (above) shows the cognitive event-related potential of a child with ADD carrying out the same task. This child, too, counted the correct number of tones, but it is clear that the P300 is not properly formed. It can be inferred that the child is having to concentrate using a less efficient attentional mechanism. Figure 5 (below) shows how the size of the P300 improves when the child is taking medicine for ADD.

The role of neuro-electrophysiological studies

Neuro-electrophysiological testing is useful because it provides objective evidence of brain immaturities and inefficiencies. It cannot be used in isolation, but forms part of the information that is required to determine whether the child has ADD or not.

Neuro-electrophysiological testing may also play an important role in determining the child's response to treatment and in reviewing the child's progress over time.

Some of the abnormalities seen on neuro-electrophysiological testing resolve when medicine for ADD is taken by the child. These changes can be used to monitor whether medicine is effective (and, in some cases, whether it is being taken). Other changes only become normal with maturity, and these can be used to decide when medicine is no longer needed.

Research is being carried out to determine whether neuro-electrophysiological data can be used to predict which particular medicine will help an individual child. There are already some patterns on neuro-electrophysiological testing that indicate that a specific medicine would be best for the child. For most children, however, medication testing as described in chapter 13 will be needed.

Neuro-electrophysiological testing can play a very important part in the diagnosis and ongoing monitoring of children with ADD. However, it is not yet widely available and many children are treated without access to this kind of evaluation.

Formulation of a management plan

Once the developmental paediatrician has collected together information about the child, a treatment plan can be developed. The paediatrician will provide a thorough explanation of the findings shortly after the examination. He or she will also make recommendations about ways of helping the child.

Parents should remember that these are only suggestions; they know their child and family best, and will need to decide whether they feel that the recommendations are right for their child and their family. If they feel unhappy with any of the suggestions, they should not hesitate to tell the paediatrician so that alternative strategies can be found.

Each treatment plan will be tailored to the child's particular areas of difficulty. There is no single approach that suits all children. Children with difficulties in a particular academic area may need remedial help, while others who are proficient in the area will not.

Medication should be considered for all children with significant difficulties, but this decision, too, needs to be individualised and depends upon the results of psychometric and neurometric testing, as well as the child's history. For example, the child who has shown rapid spontaneous improvement may not be treated if it is thought that the condition is about to resolve. A child with the same degree of difficulty, who has not shown any recent improvement and whose neuro-electrophysiological profile shows a greater degree of immaturity, may be put on to treatment.

Review assessments

If a child's problems resolve, reassessment will not be needed; however, if the child continues to have difficulties, further assessments should be carried out to monitor the child's progress and ensure that any special needs are met.

Reviews usually occur every six months and involve physical examination and psychometric and neuro-electro-physiological testing to determine how the child is progressing. A report from the child's teacher should be requested for all reviews.

Summary points

- The first step in the proper treatment of ADD is making the diagnosis.
- The best person to make the diagnosis is a developmental paediatrician working in close liaison with an educational psychologist.
- The diagnostic process involves a number of steps:
  1 A history is taken to collect information about how the child learns and behaves at home and at school.
  2 The paediatrician examines the child to ensure that there is no other condition interfering with learning and or behaviour.
  3 Psychometric testing is carried out to develop an understanding of the child's particular areas of difficulty.
  4 Neuro-electrophysiological tests provide an objective measure of brain function.
- It is then the responsibility of the paediatrician to evaluate all this information and to come to a diagnosis which he or she should explain to the parents. Recommendations can then be made about ways of helping the child.
- Reviews should usually be undertaken every six months and involve physical examination and psychometric and neuro-electrophysiological testing to determine how the child is progressing and to modify treatment where necessary.

Treatment

ten

Home management

Children with ADD are very challenging to bring up. No parent of a child with ADD will be able to respond to every difficulty that arises in a text book manner. Children with ADD often bring out the worst in their parents, and even the most patient and understanding parent is likely to make many mistakes.

All that a parent of a child with ADD should hope to achieve is to be a 'good enough' parent—a parent who tries to do his or her best, who learns from his or her mistakes, and who provides support for the child through all the difficulties that life presents.

Understanding—the first step in management

No plan of management can ever be successful if it is not based on a comprehensive assessment of the child's particular strengths and difficulties, as described in the previous chapter, and a careful explanation to both the parents, and the child, of the nature of the condition.

Unfortunately, there is a great tendency to blame any behavioural or learning difficulty on inadequacy on the part of the parents or an intentional failure on the part of the child. This belief is deeply rooted in the way in which we interpret children's behaviour. Understanding ADD requires a shift in our way of thinking about and perceiving children's actions.

We have almost lost the ability to think of the brain as an organ, just like the lungs or the heart, and to realise that its primary function is to control behaviour and learning. All behaviour is controlled by the brain.

One often hears comments such as 'His poor concentration is not due to ADD, it is behavioural!'. However, to say that a behaviour is or is not 'behavioural' is in reality meaningless. A behaviour has to be 'behavioural'—that is what that adjective means. What the person probably means by the word 'behavioural' is that the behaviour is in some way due to inadequate child rearing, or some vague notion of 'naughtiness' on the part of the child. That the word 'behavioural' has become almost synonymous with such causation tells us a great deal about how lopsided our view of the causes of children's behaviour has become.

There is no doubt that a child can behave in an unwanted way because of poor child-rearing experiences, but this is not the only, or necessarily the most common, cause of behavioural difficulties.

All unwanted behaviours in children should be looked at objectively to determine causation. Some will be due to an inadequacy in the way in which the child has been reared, many will be due to an immaturity in the child's brain, and some will be due to a mixture of the two. In other cases the cause may best be viewed as a mismatch between the child's brain and the environmental demands that are placed on her.

It is interesting that when children have difficulty walking we point to their legs as the likely cause of the problem; if they have difficulty breathing, we point to their lungs; when they have difficulty hearing we point to their ears—but when they have difficulty behaving, we point to their mothers!

Only a careful assessment can tease out the factors that relate to child rearing and those that relate to immaturities in the child's brain. Then a proper understanding and management plan can be devised.

Once it is determined that the child's difficulties are due to ADD, we must look upon the child as someone whose behaviour and learning inadequacies are due to a hidden disability that are not of her, or her parents', making. Once this is understood, the child can be helped.

Explaining to the child

Parents are sometimes concerned about telling their child that he has ADD in case he becomes upset about knowing that there is an immaturity in his brain. However, children with ADD know from an early age that there is something different about them. They know that they are getting into more trouble than other children or that they are struggling to learn things that other children are learning with ease.

Children start to compare themselves with their peers from a very early age and are quick to notice which things they find difficult. Unfortunately, if parents or professionals do not explain to the child with ADD the cause of his problems, the child is likely to come to the conclusion that he is 'dumb' or 'stupid'. Children with ADD have a tendency to find a locus of blame for things that go wrong in their lives, as described in chapter 7, and therefore can easily become angry and depressed by their difficulties.

It is therefore a good idea to tell your child about ADD at an early stage. Do not wait until he becomes confused and discouraged. Explain that different people are talented in different ways. Point out those things at which he is better, and the special qualities he has. Tell him about the things that you find difficult. Then explain that some things are very difficult for him to do, even when he tries very hard. Explain that this is simply because a part of his brain is taking a little longer to switch itself on completely.

Explain that as children grow changes occur in their bodies. They get new teeth, they grow taller, they become stronger, their bodies change into those of adults, etc. Explain that there is a little mechanism in the brain that is very important for helping a person to concentrate and control frustration and that this becomes stronger as children grow older. Describe it as being like a switch that is slowly turned on.

Just as some children get their teeth a little later, or go into puberty a little later, so in children with ADD this 'switch' takes longer to turn on completely.

Emphasise that the switch is already partly on and that the child can already concentrate and control his behaviour, but that it is far more difficult for him to do these things. You may need to explain that that is why he sometimes finds it difficult to sustain his attention, control his impulsivity, or manage to win friends.

It is important that children with ADD realise that they can do the things they find difficult, and that they are not led to believe that these things are impossible for them to achieve. However, it is essential to acknowledge the great difficulty that they experience in trying to be consistent in performing certain tasks.

There are now many good books that are written for children with ADD to explain their condition to them. These include two books written by Dr Michael Gordon: *Jumpin' Johnny Get Back To Work!* for the younger child, and *I Would If I Could* for the teenager. Jeanne Gehret has also written an excellent book for children, *Eagle Eyes—A Child's View of Attention Deficit Disorder*. Other good books include: *Shelley, The Hyperactive Turtle* (age 3–7) by Deborah Moss; *The 'Putting On The Brakes' Activity Book For Young People with ADD*, by Patricia Quinn and Judith Stern; and two books by Roberta Parker: *Making The Grade* and *Slam Dunk* which are both suitable for adolescents.

For younger children who need to take medicine for ADD, *Otto Learns About His Medicine* explains medical treatment of ADD through a story.

All books and videos recommended here can be ordered from A.D.D. WareHouse, 300 Northwest 70th Avenue, Suite 102, Plantation. FL 33317. USA. Fax: 1–305–792–8545.

Parents' needs

Before looking at ways of helping your child, it is essential to look at your own needs and concerns. Parents need help in coping with their own feelings and those of their other children, as well as other members of the family.

It is quite natural to feel guilty about your child's difficulties. Most parents report that they imagine that they are in some way to blame for the fact that their child has ADD. This may be aggravated when they find out that ADD has a very strong genetic factor to its causation and that it tends to run in families. You need to understand that ADD is due to constitutional factors within your child and is not due to anything that is under your control. Every person carries a wide variety of genes and no one can be held responsible for his or her genetic make-up. Genes, good and bad, are passed from generation to generation in a way that is beyond our control.

Because ADD runs in families, parents have often had similar difficulties to their child and this can be a double-edged sword. On the one hand, having experienced similar difficulties gives you more insight into the problems your child has faced, or may face, in the future. On the other hand, you are likely to strongly identify with your child and may find that this makes it more difficult to cope with him going through the same problems, and suffering the same hurt, that you experienced.

If you have the residual form of ADD that persists into adulthood, you will need to be aware that your own difficulties with impulsivity and rigidity might make it more difficult for you to help your child. If this is the case, you may need professional guidance to help you manage. However, parents who have had ADD do have an advantage in that they usually understand their children's difficulties in a way that a parent who did not have ADD cannot.

Parents of children with ADD experience many emotions. They may be hurt by other people's insensitive remarks about their child, they may be embarrassed by their child's difficulties, and they may feel great anxiety about how their child will cope both academically and socially. Many parents feel overwhelmed by the task of teaching their child to overcome her difficulties. They may feel angry much of the time, too—angry with teachers who fail to understand their child's problems, angry with doctors who fail to recognise their child's difficulties.

Despite these difficulties, most parents do cope and find that things become easier with time. It may be helpful to have someone to share your feelings with: a friend, a spouse, or professional, someone who will listen sympathetically and not be judgemental or too quick to offer advice.

It can be very helpful to meet other parents of a child with similar difficulties. There are now many support groups for parents of children with ADD and some of these are listed in the Appendix of this book. Support groups invite speakers who help broaden and deepen your understanding of your child's difficulties. They will also assist with strategies to manage your child.

Support groups often produce a newsletter and may have a lending library of books and videos. The greatest strengths of such groups is that they allow parents to meet informally and exchange experiences.

When a professional or other parent provides advice, you should always feel free to reject this if it does not fit in with your own child-rearing practices, or your own family's way of doing things. There is no one single right way of helping children with ADD, or of coping with the difficulties that you face. There is no single prescription that will work for everyone. Choose those things that seem right to you and fit in best with your way of doing things.

One of the most important things is to try to take one step at a time. Set yourself realistic short-term goals and concentrate on them. Try to avoid looking too far ahead. After all, your child, you, and the opportunities available to you will change in ways that cannot always be predicted.

Children with ADD cause their parents a lot of stress. It is important to find ways of reducing your own stress levels. Some parents will attend relaxation classes or stress management courses. Whenever possible find ways of recharging your own batteries. Difficulties can often be solved when you have a chance to stand back and see things in perspective.

You may also need to develop strategies for coping with other people's hurtful remarks about your child. It is worthwhile giving some thought to this so that you do not find yourself unprepared.

First, you can set an example. If someone says something inappropriate, you can simply repeat what they have said in a more appropriate way. Some parents are helped by giving themselves silent pep talks, such as 'this man doesn't know what he is talking about'.

If you know that you are going to experience a difficult but unavoidable situation, it may be worth your while rehearsing the situation before it takes place. You may do this on your own or with someone close to you. You will probably decide on a series of responses that are more appropriate than those that would have occurred without rehearsal. Sometimes such responses can be used on subsequent occasions in similar situations.

It is also important to provide information to those around you so that they understand your child's difficulties. It may be helpful to lend a book, such as this one, to a friend who does not understand your child's condition.

The needs of brothers and sisters

Siblings of a child with ADD experience special pressures. It is important that they understand the nature of ADD, that they receive attention of their own from parents, and that they develop strategies to help cope with the attitudes and comments of other children towards their brother or sister who has ADD.

You should explain to the siblings that the child with ADD is not lazy or naughty but that he has genuine difficulties in certain areas. Explain how you are trying to help him. It is important that you explain to the siblings that each child is different and that is why you have different expectations and different rules and regulations for each child. If this is explained carefully and carried out consistently, children can understand that they are not being discriminated against when it is necessary to spend more time with, or to show greater leniency towards, the child with ADD.

It is important to distinguish between disability and laziness. A child with ADD should not be able to use his disability as an excuse for quitting when a goal is attainable.

If a sibling is being teased about her brother or sister, it is important to acknowledge how hurt she must feel. Encourage her to express her anger and resentment and respond sympathetically. It is often difficult for a sibling to ignore unkind comments from her peers. It may help your child to imagine that she has an 'electric forcefield' surrounding her body that deflects any insults before they get to her.

It may be beneficial to ask the teacher to provide some help too. Sometimes a teacher can initiate a discussion about 'being different', or 'having difficulties' that may change the attitudes of other children.

The sibling of a child with ADD may also benefit from the books written for children with ADD and also some excellent videos, such as 'It's Just Attention Disorder: A video for kids', that will give him or her insight into the difficulties a child with ADD experiences. Two excellent books for siblings are *I'm Somebody Too* by Jean Geheret and *My Brother's A World Class Pain*.

Improving your child's self-esteem

Children with ADD are often very hard on themselves. They appraise themselves harshly and are quick to blame themselves for things that go wrong. As explained in chapter 7, this is partly related to immaturities in certain parts of the brain. In addition, children with ADD are often failing academically and socially. It is therefore very important that parents help children build up their self-esteem as much as possible. This is important as many of the unwanted behaviours seen in children with ADD, such as school avoidance, homework avoidance, TV addiction, cheating, aggression, controlling behaviour, bullying, quitting and depression, are maladaptive responses to low self-esteem.

The most detrimental effect of low self-esteem is that it encourages a child to enter a cycle of failure in which his ability drops lower and lower. The child tries to evade failure by avoiding challenges. This results in poor attainments that reinforce the child's feeling of inadequacy. By contrast, a child with better self-esteem will be able to try harder because he is not so frightened of failure. Because children with ADD appraise themselves so harshly, parents need to try to help their child's self-esteem.

Many a parent of a child with ADD has praised their child in the hope that this would bolster his or her self-image, only to find that the child reacted adversely to praise. The reason is that, because the child feels so inadequate, the praise reminds him of how poor his achievements are. Children with low self-esteem are often quick to misinterpret parental praise as being patronising. Some children with ADD are so insecure that they interpret praise as implied criticism or suspect that they are being compared with another child.

Yet parents need to develop their child's self-esteem. If a child with ADD has not attained good self-esteem by adulthood, she will derive little value from any other success that she attains. With high self-esteem, she will probably cope well with life, even though some difficulties persist.

How can you as parents engender high self-esteem in your child with ADD? First, you should accept your child for what she is; that is the sum total of her strengths and weaknesses. You need to see her in terms of her own uniqueness. Try to see within her the potential that she will realise at her own pace.

As parents, your role is to encourage, enjoy and value her. Try to avoid basing your own feelings of self-esteem and worth on your child's behaviour. Your child needs love that is not conditional upon her achievement. You also need to accept her feelings without criticism.

Try to emphasise her positive attributes and show how you value them. She needs plenty of praise for her efforts. However, do no overdo this or persist with praise if it clearly makes her feel uncomfortable. When praising, make it clear what you are praising her for. Avoid general comments such as, 'Well done', or 'Good girl', but rather say things such as, 'You spelt that difficult word very well', or, 'That was excellent reading'. Praise effort and not just achievement. However, when you praise effort, make it clear that it is effort you are praising. The child who tries very hard, but reads hesitantly, should be praised not for 'reading well', but for 'having a very good go'.

Children learn self-esteem from their parents' example. This is one of the reasons that children whose parents have high self-esteem are more likely to have high self-esteem themselves. You need to have faith in yourself. Let your child hear you praise your own accomplishments ('that was a job well done').

It is most important that you encourage your child to set realistic goals so that he can experience success. Help him to evaluate his achievements realistically so that he is not over-critical of himself.

It is important to set achievable goals at the start of any activity. If your child is going to attempt something that is too difficult for him, guide him to a more suitable activity in a tactful way.

You should also teach your child to praise himself. If he achieves something, ask him 'How do you think you went?'. Teach him also to praise others (for example, 'what do you think of Dad's salad?').

Children benefit from having special time with both parents. Often one parent will have little opportunity for special time. This may be because he or she is so busy with home duties and chores, or with work outside the home, that he or she never has special time with the child. Both parents should plan ways in which children will have some special time with both of them. Where parents are separated, children will have better self-esteem if they are not treated as a 'football' to be fought over by the parents. Parents owe it to their children to ensure that they work out peaceful and stable access arrangements even if this means some compromise on the part of one of the parents.

Children also need to feel that they belong to something. It may be an idea to arrange for your child to join a hobby group, a scout pack, or some other such unit. Encourage him to be proud of his school, his neighbourhood, and his ethnic tradition.

Children need to feel that they have the power to make some of the choices that affect their lives. Whenever possible, let him select things for himself, such as which clothes he wears, in what order he does things, and which books he takes from the library. Admire his choices and praise his self-sufficiency.

Another way of increasing your child's self-esteem is by enriching his experiences. Take him on excursions, teach him to do new things like gardening. Make a photo album with pictures of him. Give him opportunities to become self-reliant. Teach him to make small purchases on his own, to answer the telephone, and to take responsibility for some household task.

Your role as a teacher

Parents have an important role in helping their child to learn. They teach by example, often without realising it, and in a more direct way. For a child with ADD, the parents' role as teacher becomes even more important. No other teacher can spend as much one-to-one time with a child. No other teacher has the opportunity to extend what the child has learned in so many different situations. However, a child's relationship with her parents is generally so much more intense than with any other teacher that parents should approach teaching with care. Most parents can be good at teaching their child provided they make this a positive and constructive experience for the child. This means that the parent must be prepared to put some thought into how to become an effective teacher.

Before you teach your child, you should liaise with her class teacher. He or she will ensure that what you teach complements what is being done at school. A good teacher will be happy to give you guidance about what to teach and how to go about it. He or she will be only too aware that there is usually insufficient time to give adequate individual tuition to each child in the class.

When you teach your child, do not overdo it. Short daily sessions are much better than infrequent long sessions. Attempt small units of work at a time. Do ensure that you are teaching your child the things that she is learning at school. You do not want to add to her burden by increasing the amount she has to learn. Aim to make those things that she already has to do at school easier.

Choose a time when you are both feeling calm. You need a quiet environment where you will not be disturbed. It may be necessary for you to arrange for your other children to be occupied somewhere else. Do not have a teaching session when you are doing something else, while the TV is on, or when siblings are around.

Try to make sessions as enjoyable and as varied as possible. Start with a revision of the previous work, and explain what you hope to achieve in this session and why it is important. Work slowly and patiently. Sometimes your child will seem to have a block or forget things that she knew the previous day. Take this in your stride. It is perfectly normal for children to progress slowly, with sudden spurts followed by protracted periods of comparatively little progress. During these slow phases children are often consolidating skills before going on to the next stage.

Because children with ADD have to work so hard to concentrate, you may need to have frequent breaks. Some children benefit from having a chance to burn off excess energy before they start work. Other children will become so excited by physical activity that they then find it difficult to settle down to do homework afterwards. Children with ADD who have difficulty in focusing after intense physical activity may be better working first and engaging in physical activities later.

The timing of the child's medication is very important with regard to when it is best to do homework or study. For example, a child who takes dexamphetamine or Ritalin (methylphenidate) in the afternoon should probably start working approximately one hour after the tablet has been taken. In this way she will be most settled when needed.

When working with your child, always be encouraging, never critical. Avoid expressions such as 'Hurry up', 'Watch what you're doing', 'Don't be careless', and 'You have seen that word before'. Instead, use phrases such as 'You are really improving at reading', and 'You really worked hard on this'.

Whenever you have a teaching session with your child, end it with an activity that she is good at and enjoys. At the end, do not forget to say something like 'That was fun, I look forward to doing some more with you tomorrow'. When the session is over, try to stop playing the part of the teacher. You are more than a teacher, you are a parent as well. Parents cannot treat every interaction with their child as an opportunity for teaching without the relationship becoming stilted and the child becoming resentful. There must be opportunities for unstructured interaction.

Teaching has to concentrate on the child's areas of weakness. Most children are aware from an early age of things they find difficult. Like the rest of us, they want to spend time on the things they are better at. Make certain that you give your child ample opportunities to do those things that she is good at, in addition to those she finds difficult. This is essential for her self-confidence.

Some parents do not have the time or the ability to teach their child. In this case, it is usually best to find a teacher or coach to help your child after school. It is important to choose someone with the skills and temperament to do this well. Support organisations often have lists of suitable teachers. The names of some of these organisations can be found in the Appendix.

Working with the school

It is best to regard yourself, the teachers, and other professionals (such as speech therapists) involved with your child's education as a team. Each member of the team plays a part in providing the best education for the child. It is essential that you and the other members of the team communicate regularly.

Some schools have a file for each child which is passed on to his new teacher every year. Do not rely on this, but arrange a meeting with your child's new teacher at the beginning of each year. At the meeting explain your child's difficulties and give the teacher copies of any assessments done in the past.

During the year, keep in regular contact with the teacher to find out how your child is progressing. It is a good idea for the child's homework diary to be used as a 'communication book' in which you and the teacher can exchange information on a regular basis. You should not hesitate to request a special meeting with your child's teacher if there is something causing you concern. Do this as early as possible.

It is sometimes possible to apply for funding for special teaching sessions at school for a child with ADD. These may be given in the class or in a resource room. The child may receive individual help, or be part of a small group of children with similar difficulties. If you think this may be possible, check with your child's teacher to see whether it is available. Some schools have an arrangement whereby parents come to the class and help children with their reading or other work.

Try not to become involved in discipline issues that should be the domain of the school. If a child is misbehaving at school, the teachers, possibly with the aid of the principal, should develop strategies for dealing with this. The school may need to call upon a psychologist attached to the school if such expert advice is needed.

As a parent, it is probably best if you are not put in the position of having to punish your child for misdemeanours at school. This only increases stresses at home and creates negative interactions between parent and child. While you should always be prepared to go to the school at the teacher's request to discuss behavioural problems, you should try wherever possible to encourage the school to deal with these problems, while you deal with the behaviour problems you observe at home. Often the best role for a parent of a child who is behaving badly at school is to provide him with a happy home environment where he is given unconditional love. In this way behaviour at school may improve as the child's self-esteem is built up.

Summary points

- All that a parent of a child with ADD should hope to achieve is to be a 'good enough' parent—a parent who tries to do his or her best, who learns from his or her mistakes and who supports the child through all the difficulties that life presents.
- No plan of management will be successful if it is not based on a comprehensive assessment of the child's particular strengths and difficulties and a careful explanation, to both the parents and the child, of the nature of the condition.
- Unfortunately, if parents or professionals do not explain to the child with ADD the cause of his problems, the child is likely to come to the conclusion that he is 'dumb' or 'stupid'.
- It is important for the child with ADD to realise that he *can* do the things that he finds difficult. However, it is essential to acknowledge the great difficulty that he experiences in trying to be consistent in performing certain tasks.
- It may be helpful to have someone to share your feelings with: a friend, a spouse, or professional; someone who will listen sympathetically and not be judgemental or too quick to offer advice.
- It can be very helpful to meet other parents of a child with similar difficulties.

- Siblings of a child with ADD experience special pressures. It is important that they understand the nature of ADD, that they receive attention of their own from parents, and that they develop strategies to help cope with the attitudes and comments of other children towards the brother or sister who has ADD.
- Accept your child for what she is; that is the sum total of her strengths and weaknesses. You need to see her in terms of her own uniqueness. Try to see within her the potential that she will realise at her own pace.
- When praising, make it clear what you are praising her for. Praise effort and not just achievement.
- No other teacher can spend as much one-to-one time with a child as a parent. No other teacher has the opportunity to extend what the child has learned in so many different situations.
- Before you teach your child, you should liaise with her class teacher.
- When you teach your child, do not overdo it. Short daily sessions are better than infrequent long sessions. Choose a time when you are both calm. Have frequent breaks. Arrange for medication to be working during teaching sessions.
- Arrange a meeting with your child's new teacher at the beginning of each year to explain your child's difficulties.
- Try not to become involved in discipline issues that should be the domain of the school.

eleven

School management

The average school-age child spends well over a third of his time in school. A child's experiences in the classroom, and in the playground, will affect his academic attainments, the development of his self-esteem, and his social skills. Since these are the areas where children with ADD have difficulties, it is essential that teachers and principals understand how best to help children with this common disability.

In the past, teachers often had little understanding of the needs of a child with ADD. Such children were labelled as 'lazy' or 'bad', and often dealt with harshly. Problems with learning and social skills were not detected early and children were not assessed adequately. Parents were often blamed for their child's difficulties. Those parents who arranged for their children's difficulty to be properly assessed and diagnosed often found that teachers and principals had never heard of ADD. Educational programmes were not implemented and the school could be uncooperative with medication regimes.

Now there is a growing awareness of ADD within the education system. Teachers are increasingly being taught about ADD in their university training and in-service courses. Many State education departments have produced guidelines and information booklets about ADD for teaching staff.

The interested teacher can also gain access to a number of books written especially for teachers about ADD. These include books such as *The ADD Hyperactivity Handbook for Schools* by Harvey C. Parker and *Attention Without Tension: A Teacher's Handbook on Attention Disorders* by Copeland and Love. These are books written for teachers by specialist teachers and psychologists. There are also many videos that give an insight into appropriate teaching techniques. These include 'Educating Inattentive Children', by Samuel and Michael Goldstein, and 'ADHD in the Classroom: Strategies for Teachers', by Russell Barkley. For teachers who want to understand how best to help a child with ADD, there are now many sources of information and special teaching materials. All these books, videos, and teaching materials may be ordered from the ADDWareHouse.

Unfortunately, there are still teachers who are ignorant of ADD. Many of these teachers will be eager to become informed about ADD when they realise that they have a child in their class with it. Other teachers, a decreasing minority, will claim that they 'do not believe in ADD', or that they are 'against' certain treatments such as medication. Such teachers may prefer to blame parents for the child's difficulties, claim that the child is lazy, or believe that punishing the child will remedy the problem. They may have misconceptions about the role of medication in this disorder and be ignorant of the literature on ADD. Some have a misconception that all children with ADD are constantly active, and do not understand the wide range of difficulties seen in children with this condition.

Which school?

Choosing a child's school usually requires some degree of compromise on the part of the parents. Whatever placement you eventually decide upon, it is unlikely to be perfect. Schools rarely are. What you need to find is the best alternative for your child at that stage of her education. Always keep in mind that no placement needs to be permanent. Regular reviews should be undertaken, and your child could move to a more appropriate class or school if her needs are found to have changed.

All things being equal, a child is usually best placed at a school that is near to her home. Beside making transportation easier, it also gives the child an opportunity to meet and mix with neighbourhood children with whom she will be able to play after school.

It is essential that the principal of the school has a good understanding of ADD. This means that he or she should know about the condition, have an enlightened attitude towards comprehensive assessment, and be prepared to implement a multimodal treatment plan which includes behaviour management, special educational help, and medication. If the principal does not understand ADD, it is going to be extremely difficult to ensure that the child receives appropriate help.

The classes in the school should preferably not be too large. It is very difficult for one teacher to help a child with ADD if there are more than 30 children in the class. Classrooms should be closed spaces (not open plan). Seating should be in rows with children facing the teacher, rather than with desks placed in small clusters.

The school should be structured with clear-cut rules which children can understand. School programs that allow children to come and go as they please and to choose which activities they want to take part in are often not appropriate for children with ADD.

Children should be in classes grouped by age so that they have a feeling of belonging with their peer group. Composite classes and 'vertical streaming' systems are usually confusing and distracting for most children with ADD.

It is best if children are streamed according to ability for each individual subject. This allows children who are weaker in a particular subject to receive extra help and to work at an appropriate pace. It also enables a child to have the satisfaction of moving up to a higher stream as she improves.

The school should employ support teachers for children with learning difficulties so that they can receive extra help within the ordinary class.

The classroom teacher should understand ADD and be able to implement the strategies discussed below for helping children who are experiencing difficulties.

Effective strategies for teaching children with ADD

Diagnosis and assessment first

It is essential that a child who is experiencing difficulties in the classroom or the playground should first have an adequate assessment before any management plan is formulated. Such an assessment involves a developmental paediatrician and psychologist as discussed in chapter 9.

No management plan should be devised until such an assessment has been carried out to establish the child's particular strengths and difficulties and to identify the cause or causes of the child's problems.

Teachers' attitudes

To properly manage a child with ADD, a teacher must have an understanding of what it is like to be a child with ADD. The teacher should also have some insight into his or her own make-up and response to the child. Some teachers have a natural ability to empathise with children who have ADD, and find it easy to get the best out of such children. Other teachers may find that they become very angry and frustrated with children with ADD and that their natural teaching style, which may be successful with children who do not have this condition, is not suitable for children with ADD.

A teacher who feels frustrated by the difficulties presented by a child with ADD, who finds it difficult to carry out a behaviour management programme or make classroom adjustments for the child with ADD, should turn to the school psychologist. With regular consultation with the psychologist, the teacher should be able to gain insight into his or her difficulties and develop better strategies for overcoming these.

Classroom accommodation

It is important that the teacher should create a proper learning environment for the child with ADD. The child with ADD should be seated in the front of the class near to the teacher's desk. The teacher should ensure that the child's seat is part of the regular class seating and not separate from the other children. By placing her at the front, the teacher can ensure that he or she has the child's attention. This position also has the advantage that the child with ADD will have her back to the rest of the class so that other students are less likely to distract her. It can thus be seen that the old idea of putting the 'naughty' child at the back of the class, or letting such a child seat herself at the back of the class, is totally inappropriate if the child has ADD.

It is a good idea to place children who will serve as good role models on either side of the child with ADD. Example is the greatest teacher and the child with ADD will benefit from copying the behaviour of the children around her, and will also be less distracted by them if they are well-behaved and have good work habits. The teacher can make the most of the proximity of these good role models by encouraging peer teaching and cooperative learning.

Wherever possible, the teacher should keep the child with ADD away from distracting stimuli. The child should be seated well away from distractions such as an air-conditioner or window.

Children with ADD do need to be in an interesting environment, but the teacher should avoid creating a learning environment that is too 'busy'. Rather than filling the classroom with posters covered with information, and objects such as mobiles, the teacher should aim to make the classroom interesting but muted in tone. School bags should be placed at the back of the class out of the way, and the desks and boards should be kept uncluttered.

The playground

In the same way that it is important to provide an appropriate learning environment for the child in the classroom, it is important that the child with ADD be adequately catered for in the playground.

Children with ADD often need supervision in the playground so that they do not cause problems to themselves or others. This supervision should be carried out in such a way that the child with ADD does not feel he is being singled out.

If the child with ADD wishes to play with younger children in the playground, this should be allowed. Often children with ADD have more in common with younger children and feel happiest in that social setting. Provided that they are not causing any disruption or harm, they should be allowed to play with any child.

If a child with ADD is having difficulties getting on with other children, it is useful to arrange for the school psychologist to talk to him about effective strategies for getting on with other children. It may be very difficult for the child with ADD to apply these strategies, but such intervention may pay great dividends.

Children with ADD usually benefit from individualised activities that are non-competitive. Many do not do well in team sports. The child may be encouraged to take part in games such as t-ball and trampoline if these suit him well.

Working with parents as a team

The teacher of a child with ADD should keep in regular contact with the child's parents. Sometimes this is best done through a communication book or the child's school diary. For confidential matters, a special meeting should be arranged.

The aim of the parent–teacher communication is to ensure that everyone is aware of how the child is progressing and what steps are being taken to help the child in the school and home environments. It also gives teachers an opportunity to speak to parents about ways of helping the child with his work at home. Teachers can encourage parents to help the child with his study and to review completed homework. It also allows the teacher to suggest whether remedial help is needed after school.

Parents can play a role in ensuring that their child's books and bag are organised and that particular difficulties with homework are conveyed to the teacher.

Parents should not have to punish children for misdemeanours at school. Parents should also not have to punish children for homework that is not done. Although many educators favour what is known as 'a home and school based contingency programme' (where the parents administer rewards and consequences at home, based upon a teacher's assessment), such programmes are inappropriate for most, if not all, children with ADD.

There are a number of drawbacks to home and school based contingency programmes. First, children with ADD have a lot of difficulty delaying gratification long enough to receive rewards at home for behaviour at school. Second, it seems inappropriate that a child who has been well-behaved at home, but had a bad day at school, should be punished by his parents. By rights, parents should, in this situation, be rewarding the child for his good home behaviour. Third, children with ADD are unreliable about bringing teacher's report cards home. A further problem with such programmes is that, because parents are not present at school, they are at a great disadvantage if the child wants to defend his actions at school. Parents cannot be sure whether the behaviour was misinterpreted, misunderstood, or was a reasonable response to provocation. It is, therefore, the teacher's role to monitor behaviour at school and to deal with this appropriately.

Giving instructions

Children with ADD have poor listening skills and it is important that teachers understand how to give instructions to their students with ADD.

First it is important to gain the child's attention. It is usually necessary to stand in front of the child, and even to touch the child, in order to ensure that she is able to listen to you. Do not insist that the child looks at you, however, as children with ADD often have low self-esteem and find it difficult to maintain eye contact. To force the child to look at you may only make her feel extremely uncomfortable so that she is unable to concentrate on what you are saying. Unfortunately, some teachers regard a child's failure to look at them as rudeness and punish such children. Teachers should not say things such as, 'Look at me when I am talking to you!' to a child with ADD. Children who avert their gaze, or look downwards, may not be rude at all: simply embarrassed and uncomfortable.

The instructions should be as brief and clear as possible. Avoid giving instructions that contain a number of different parts, such as 'Go to the back of the class, open your bag, and take out your maths book!'. It would be more appropriate to simply say 'Go to your bag', and then, only when the child is at her bag, to say 'Take out your maths book'. Children with ADD have problems with short-term memory and find it very difficult to retain a two- or three-part instruction.

It is always important to ensure that the child understands an instruction before beginning the task. It may be necessary to repeat the instruction. This should be done in a friendly, calm manner.

Unfortunately, many children with ADD do not ask for help and a teacher should always try to create an environment where the child with ADD will feel comfortable seeking assistance.

Children with ADD often have difficulty carrying out instructions because of their poor organisation skills. It may be necessary for children to have all books for a particular subject colour coded. They may need a list of the steps required to carry out instructions.

It is essential that teachers ensure that the child is supervised when writing down his homework and that parents know how to check this work. A child with ADD who is asked to do a task should have regular monitoring to ensure that he knows what is expected and whether he is succeeding.

With all instructions, the teacher should ensure that the child is actually capable of carrying out the task and that it is not beyond his abilities.

Modifying work and examinations for the child with ADD

Teachers should ensure that children with ADD are tested on their knowledge and not unfairly penalised for their difficulties with concentration.

It is important not to overload the child with tasks that need a great deal of persistence. For example, it may be necessary to shorten the work so that the child only does every second mathematics problem.

When setting out questions for the child, these should be given in 'bite size' sections, rather than giving the child a page filled with questions. The tasks should be broken up into smaller stages, each one on a separate piece of paper; each sheet is then given to the child separately.

It may be important for the teacher to consult with the school counsellor, or special education teacher, to modify assignments and homework according to the child's particular areas of strength and weakness. The development of an individualised education programme for the child may be necessary.

It may be best to give the child extra time to finish examinations. Children with ADD are easily frustrated and do poorly under the stress of an examination. They also find it very difficult to write down their thoughts on paper and usually do better in a multiple choice examination than in the essay type.

In any examination, it is important that the teacher be available to answer queries. Children with ADD are less likely to seek assistance and it may be important for the teacher to keep an eye on what the child is doing in a discreet way, so as to be able to guide the child if she has misunderstood the question.

Behaviour management

In the next chapter behaviour modification for parents is described. Teachers can implement the same sort of programmes with children who have specific behaviours that are causing difficulties.

It is essential that a teacher be able to talk to a child with ADD in private, in order to discuss ways in which the child may be helped. The teacher should be able to take the child aside in a way that is not obvious to the other children in the class and be able to discuss areas of behaviour that are a problem. This should be done calmly so that child and teacher can develop some strategies together. Clear consequences for misbehaviour should be established from the outset. The methods of monitoring the behaviour should be discussed. Discipline should always be appropriate to the misdemeanour and not unnecessarily harsh. Reasonable allowance should also be made for periods of difficulty.

It should always be remembered that children with ADD manage transitions very poorly and some allowance should be made for this. Such transitions include periods when they come into the classroom after breaks, when they move from one classroom to another, or when they have a new teacher. They are liable to become over-excited when they are due to have some activity that they enjoy, such as an outing or a sports event, and this should also be taken into consideration.

In all situations, the teacher should aim to help the child's self-esteem. Ridicule and criticism should always be avoided. Rewards should be used liberally in order to help build up the child's self-esteem. Rewards should be given as soon as possible after wanted behaviour has been demonstrated. Teach the child to reward herself by encouraging positive self-talk ('You finished the job very well. How do you feel about that?'). This sort of cognitive re-structuring encourages the child to be more positive about herself.

Wherever possible try to encourage the child to monitor herself. This teaches her self-control. Self-monitoring requires that the student observes her own behaviour and records the observations. For example, a child can be given a check list in which she is asked to mark whether she was paying attention whenever she hears a beep on a tape. A commercially available programme, 'The Listen, Look and Think Program' (Impact

Publications Inc.), is available. It is helpful for the student to compare her ratings with those of the teacher.

Extra help for children with ADD

Children with ADD are often behind in one or more areas of academic attainments. They may therefore need some individualised help. Children with ADD usually learn very well in a one-to-one situation and may make rapid strides if given some individualised attention.

Teachers may be able to find time during the school day when they can sit down with the child and provide help on a one-to-one basis. If this is not available, or if the teacher cannot provide sufficient help in this way, it is important to look for other ways of giving the child such assistance.

Schools may be able to fund a special needs teacher who provides help on a one-to-one basis to children with learning difficulties. If this is not available, the teacher should consider whether a volunteer can provide this kind of help. Such volunteers may be parents or senior citizens. A good teacher will know how to utilise a volunteer in the classroom. This may be through training the volunteer to give one-to-one help, or by letting the volunteer take over some other chore so that the teacher can spend more individual time with the child who has ADD. Volunteers do need to be trained and supervised and should be treated in a professional manner. They need to be made aware that all information pertaining to a student must be treated in a confidential manner.

When children are clearly unable to receive sufficient help for their difficulties in the classroom, teachers should advise parents to arrange for extra help outside of school hours. With so many children in most classes, it is often necessary for children with learning difficulties to receive help from a tutor on a regular basis after school. It is best if the classroom teacher ensures that such help is appropriate.

The teacher may be able to recommend an appropriate tutor. He or she should be prepared to meet with the tutor to ensure that work in the classroom can be reinforced by the tutor. It is essential that the tutor should make the child's school work easier for him, and not add extra or different work for the child to do.

The teacher and the child's medication

Teachers have an important role in supervising the administration of medication for children with ADD and in monitoring the positive, as well as the negative, effects of such medication. In order to do this effectively, the teacher should understand the important role that medication plays in helping children with ADD. The teacher who is ignorant about the potential advantages of medication in such children will not be able to take on this role.

The teacher should understand that medication is one of the components of helping the child. It is to be used together with other strategies in order to get the best results.

It is important that children who take medication for ADD should not feel self-conscious about this. Teachers should never remind students publicly to take their medicine. In some cases children are able to supervise the administration of their medication on their own, and teachers need play no part in the actual administration. For younger and less capable children, the teacher may need to ensure, in a discreet way, that the child takes his tablet. In all schools children take medication regularly for conditions such as asthma, and it should be quite usual for children to take medicine in the classroom, or to go up to one of the staff rooms to take medication. Teachers should ensure that this can happen without any fuss.

The taking of medication should never be alluded to at other times. Certainly, a teacher should not comment on the child's performance in relation to whether medication has been taken or not.

Teachers and principals are often concerned about a child having medicine in his possession. They are concerned that some other child may get hold of the medicine and take it. First, it is not necessary for a child to have in his possession at school more than a single dose of the medicine. This is usually the tablet taken at recess or lunch. It is extremely unlikely that another child would take this tablet, but if one did, no harm would come to the other child. A single dose of any of the medicines taken for ADD would be safer than taking a single dose of almost any other medicine used in paediatrics (including aspirin). Children should be taught from an early age not to take other people's tablets.

Teachers also have the important role of monitoring the effects of medication. There are now a number of check-lists that teachers can use to tick off the effects of medication that they observe. Teachers are well placed to notice effects, both good and bad, that result from medication.

Table 4 shows a rating scale which teachers can use for this purpose. If untoward reactions are noted by the teacher, he or she should convey this to the parents. With the parents' permission it may be necessary for the paediatrician and teacher to discuss the effects of the medication so that the dose can be adjusted.

Sometimes, children with ADD show an improvement in their concentration at the expense of becoming slightly subdued by the medication. In consultation with the teacher, the paediatrician can lower the dosage so that the positive effect on concentration remains, while the subduing effect of the medication disappears.

It is unfortunate that there are still many teachers and principals who are negative about medicine for ADD. Because of this attitude, paediatricians and parents may decide not to involve the teacher in monitoring the child's medication. They may even decide not to tell the teacher that the child is taking medication for fear that he or she will react in a negative way and make the child feel uncomfortable about his treatment. In such a situation, the teacher is doing the child a great disservice. Such teachers, are, by their attitudes, disqualifying themselves from playing an important role in a vital aspect of their pupil's education.

Table 4   Medication effects rating scale

Behaviour	Never	Occasionally	Appropriate for age
Attentive to teacher	_____	_____	_____
Persistent with work	_____	_____	_____
Inconsistent work	_____	_____	_____
Neat work	_____	_____	_____
Disruptive in class	_____	_____	_____
Accepted by peers	_____	_____	_____
Carries out instructions	_____	_____	_____
Follows routines	_____	_____	_____
Tantrums	_____	_____	_____
Stays in seat	_____	_____	_____
Rude to teacher	_____	_____	_____
Remembers work	_____	_____	_____
Tries hard	_____	_____	_____
Negative comments about self	_____	_____	_____
Obeys rules	_____	_____	_____

Side effects	Never	Mild	Severe
Staring into space	_____	_____	_____
Abnormally subdued	_____	_____	_____
Sad	_____	_____	_____
Anxious	_____	_____	_____
Headaches	_____	_____	_____
Abdominal pain	_____	_____	_____
Rebound	_____	_____	_____
Tics	_____	_____	_____

Summary points

- There is a growing awareness of ADD within the education system. Teachers are increasingly being taught about ADD in their university training and in in-service courses. Many State education departments have started to produce guidelines and information booklets about ADD for teaching staff.
- The choice of an appropriate school is essential. The principal of the school should have a good understanding of

ADD. The classes in the school should ideally not be large. The school should be structured with clear-cut rules.

- It is essential that a child who is experiencing difficulties in the classroom or playground should first have an adequate assessment before any management plan is formulated.

- To properly manage a child with ADD, a teacher should have an understanding of what it is like to be a child with ADD. A teacher who feels frustrated by the difficulties that a child with ADD presents, who finds it difficult to carry out behaviour management programmes or make classroom adjustments for the child, should turn to the school psychologist for help.

- It is important that the teacher should create a proper learning environment for the child with ADD. The child should be seated in the front of the class near to the teacher's desk. Children who will serve as good role models should be placed on either side of the child with ADD. Wherever possible, the teacher should keep the child away from distracting stimuli. The teacher should avoid creating a learning environment that is too 'busy'.

- Children with ADD often need supervision in the playground so that they do not cause problems to themselves or others. This supervision should be done in such a way that it seems to apply to all children, in order that the child with ADD should not feel singled out.

- If a child with ADD is having difficulties getting on with other children, it is useful to arrange for the school psychologist to talk to him about effective strategies for getting on with other children. The psychologist may supervise small social skills groups.

- The teacher of a child with ADD should keep in regular contact with the child's parents. Sometimes this is best done through a communication book or the child's school diary. When it is important that the child should not be aware of what is being discussed, a special meeting should be arranged.

- Parents should not have to punish children for misdemeanours at school. Parents should also not have to punish children for homework that is not done. It is the teacher's role to monitor behaviour at school and to deal with this appropriately.

- Children with ADD have poor listening skills and it is important that teachers understand how to give instructions to these students.

- Many children with ADD do not ask for help and a teacher should always try to create an environment where the child with ADD will feel comfortable seeking assistance.

- Teachers should ensure that children with ADD are tested on their knowledge and not penalised for their difficulties with concentration.

- It is essential that a teacher should be able to talk to a child with ADD in private, to discuss ways in which the child may be helped.

- It should always be remembered that children with ADD manage transitions very poorly and some allowance should be made for this.

- In all situations, the teacher should aim to build up the child's self-esteem. Ridicule and criticism should always be avoided. Rewards should be used liberally in order to help build up the child's self-esteem. Rewards should be given as soon as possible after desirable behaviour has been observed.

- Teachers should teach the child with ADD to reward herself by encouraging positive self-talk.

- Children with ADD are often behind in one or more areas of academic attainments. They may therefore need some individualised help from a tutor, a special needs teacher, or a volunteer.

- Teachers have an important role in supervising the administration of medication for children with ADD, and in monitoring the positive as well as the negative effects of such medication.

twelve

Behaviour modification

Behaviour modification is a form of teaching that is employed in situations where explanation alone does not succeed. Most parents practise behaviour modification without realising it. They do this by rewarding their child for good behaviour and punishing her for bad. Some parents need help in order to do this in the most effective way. Children benefit from knowing where they stand, and being able to direct their energies into more constructive and rewarding activities.

Step 1—Identify the behaviour

The first step in a behaviour modification programme is to observe your child's behaviour and identify the behaviour you want to change. You need to avoid general statements about your child such as 'she is impossible', and instead focus on specific things she does that worry or annoy you, for instance not getting dressed in the morning, or fighting with a sibling.

Step 2—What kind of behaviour is it?

There are two kinds of behaviour: good behaviour, which you want to encourage, and undesirable behaviour, which you want to get rid of. In the above examples, the good behaviour you want to encourage is getting dressed in the morning and the undesirable behaviour you want to get rid of is fighting with the sibling. Ideally, it is always best to teach a child a useful skill to replace an unwanted behaviour. For example, if a child is fighting with siblings, try to think of an alternative behaviour that the child can become involved in to replace this.

Step 3—Examine antecedents and consequences

This way of looking at behaviour is sometimes known as the 'ABC' method. 'A' is for antecedents, which are those triggers that encourage unwanted behaviour. 'B' stands for the behaviour, which needs to be carefully defined. 'C' stands for the consequences, i.e. those things that happen because of the behaviour. It is important to work out which particular consequences maintain a behaviour, i.e. what keeps the child behaving in this particular way.

In the above example, if every time the child with ADD hits her sibling she receives attention from the parent, even if this attention is not good quality attention (such as shouting), this may reward and reinforce the behaviour. Children enjoy attention, and if the only sort of attention they can get is negative attention, they will still continue behaving in such a way as to receive it.

Encouraging good behaviour so that it can be rewarded

It is important to encourage desirable behaviour which can then be rewarded. Often children with ADD demonstrate so little desirable behaviour that parents have difficulty finding something that they can reward. Medication may play an important role in this regard in that children may only start behaving in a desirable way once they are on medication.

One way of encouraging good behaviour is to demonstrate the behaviour to the child in the hope he will imitate it. Some children seem more keen to imitate behaviour than others.

Your child may copy the parent he identifies with more strongly, and you should take advantage of this. For example, if you want your child to sit down and do homework it may be best if the father sits down to do his work and invites the child to sit at the same table and join him. Children also tend to copy other children. It is useful to encourage your child to come into contact with good role models whom he may imitate.

Another way of encouraging good behaviour is by modifying the child's environment. If a child takes a long time to dress, ensure his clothes are set out so that they are easy to put on, that the room is warm, and that there are minimal distractions.

If, as sometimes happens, the correct behaviour suddenly occurs, you should take advantage of this and reward the child immediately. Be alert to 'catch' your child demonstrating a good behaviour so that this can be rewarded.

How to reward good behaviour

How should you reward your child? The simplest sort of reward would be to praise what the child has done by making a fuss, smiling, and saying 'well done', or 'quick dressing', or 'good reading' etc.

Note that 'good' is used to describe the behaviour, not the child. This emphasises what you are praising, and does not in any way reflect on the child's worth. These simple verbal rewards should always be given and are often more powerful than parents realise. In some cases, however, they are not enough on their own. The older the child, the less likely that this simple kind of reward will suffice. In this case, you need to provide some tangible reward. This may take the form of a star on a chart, a 'smiley' stamp on the hand, a sweet, a raisin, a special toy, or an outing. With more sophisticated children, it may be necessary to have a system where a specific number of small tokens earns something a little larger.

Beware of the trap of making the reward too big or too expensive. You should not make it too easy to get big rewards, although you should make it reasonably easy to earn lesser rewards to encourage the child.

Sometimes a reward system is best run along the lines of a 'response–cost' system where the child forfeits some tokens when unwanted behaviour occurs.

Children with ADD often benefit from a system where they initially receive all the tokens for the week, or day, so that they can see the reward from the outset. They then have to give up a certain number of tokens that they have in their possession whenever they display unwanted behaviour. This works well because children with ADD experience difficulty working towards a reward that will only become available to them at some future time.

In all cases stamps, tokens, or charts should be available at the outset. Once the behaviour modification programme is in operation, you will need to revise the reward system if it is clear that the child is waiting too long for a reward, or is getting too many rewards.

Keep up this tangible reward system until the child loses interest, which he will invariably do once the desired behaviour has been established for a period of time. Do keep up the praise, however, even when tangible rewards are no longer given.

How to discourage undesirable behaviour

Discouraging undesirable behaviour causes parents much difficulty and confusion. Without realising it, they often reward the bad behaviour, or use ineffective ways of eradicating unwanted behaviour.

The most common *ineffective* method is to scold the child or to argue with her. Most parents would agree that this is not usually successful. The reason is that, for many children, any attention from their parent acts as a reward. Children thrive on attention, and always seem to want more. They prefer praise, but any attention, even scolding, can be rewarding for a child. (A good analogy for this is that children usually like crisp potato chips; however, if only soggy potato chips are available, they will usually eat them.)

Some parents resort to smacking their child, but usually find that this does not help for long. This may make parents very distressed, as they regard smacking as the most extreme action they can take. The reason why smacking does not seem to work is probably because it *is* such an extreme thing to do. Although it is unpleasant for the child, it is also unpleasant for the parent and most children realise this. After the smack, parents invariably feel guilty; when the pain caused by the smack has subsided, the child may enjoy the sympathy he senses from the remorseful parent. Smacking may therefore work for the moment, but usually does not eradicate a recurrent behaviour.

Pretending to ignore

What can parents do when these traditional methods do not work? Parents may need to learn that often the best thing to do is *to do nothing*. Children thrive on attention, even in the form of shouting and smacking. By withholding attention, many behaviours will diminish or disappear. Ignoring behaviour is a difficult thing to do; in fact it is questionable whether parents can ever completely ignore their child's behaviour. You can, however, *pretend* to ignore the behaviour if it is not too dangerous or disruptive. To do this you have to stifle your natural responses, avoid making eye contact with the child, and look calm. Busy yourself with some activity unrelated to the child and refuse to become involved in any discussion or argument about the behaviour that you are trying to eradicate. When the child has stopped demonstrating the particular behaviour, invite him to take part in what you are doing and resume normal conversation with him. Do not show annoyance once you start interacting with him again.

Time-out

In the case of behaviours which are too destructive, or possibly dangerous, you cannot pretend to ignore your child because of the concern that she may injure herself, or damage something or someone. You may be so angry with her that you may be afraid of losing control and harming her. In such situations, you have to remove the child to a place where she can no longer receive the reward of your attention.

This technique is known as 'time-out', and consists of insisting that the child stay on her own for a while. The aim of using 'time-out' is not to create discomfort or fear in the child but simply to remove her from the place where she is receiving reinforcement for what she is doing. Usually the most convenient place for 'time-out' is a child's bedroom. Leave her there until you have both calmed down. While the child is there, any shouting or screaming should be ignored.

It is important not to allow the child out until she has quietened down, otherwise she may get the idea that she has been allowed out because of her screaming and shouting. You can either tell the child in a calm voice that you will not allow her out until she is quiet, or if she does not understand this and will not cooperate, you can wait until there is a pause in her crying and then allow her out.

Some children are so destructive in their own room that it may be necessary to pick another room in the house. Concern is sometimes expressed that, if a child spends 'time-out' in her bedroom, she will develop a bad association with it. In practice this does not seem to occur.

At the end of a period of 'time-out', do not demand apology or engage in recriminations. Be friendly and matter of fact.

One should never use 'time-out' without giving some thought to the quality of interaction that you have with the child when you are together. In other words, one should not only be thinking of 'time-out', but also of 'time-in'. Wherever possible you should try to ensure that the time your child spends with you promotes positive interactions and encourages wanted behaviour. You do not need to continually entertain your child or spoil her during the time she is with you. However, you need to ensure that she is getting sufficient quality time with you so that she is not forced to get your attention through undesirable behaviour.

It is very easy for an exhausted and stressed parent to find that they are not giving their child good quality 'time-in'.

Quality time simply implies that you are giving your child your undivided attention and that both of you are enjoying yourselves.

Brief restraint

In situations where 'time-out' cannot be used, another way of managing aggressive behaviour is to firmly hold the child's arm at his sides for a count of fifteen. He is then released. If the behaviour recurs, this should be repeated. This method is known as 'brief restraint'. It is not suitable for a child who is physically stronger than the parent.

When holding a child in brief restraint, you should not interact with him. The idea is to stop the pleasure of walking and running about for a few minutes, not make the restraint itself a form of positive interaction.

Extinction

There are some situations where a child becomes used to being rewarded for an unwanted behaviour. An example is prolonged calling out at night which eventually results in the desired parent's appearance in the room. The withdrawal of such a reward is called 'extinction'.

There are two ways of doing this: abrupt withdrawal or gradual withdrawal. The latter is sometimes referred to as 'controlled crying' and is usually favoured. In this method, you need to wait for longer and longer periods before returning to your child. The attention given to the child on your return should be minimal.

With extinction, you should be prepared for the behaviour to worsen initially. This usually lasts a few days, and if you hold firm, the behaviour will rapidly diminish and disappear. After a variable period, there is often a reappearance of the behaviour, as if your child is testing whether the new rules still apply. If you continue to be consistent, the behaviour will cease.

Before embarking on an extinction programme, both the parents should prepare themselves for a trying time. During the period when the behaviour worsens, it is important to support one another.

Important considerations in a behaviour modification plan

Behaviour modification is straightforward in theory— encourage and reward good behaviour, discourage bad. In practice it can be very difficult, particularly as children reach adolescence.

First you should always take into account the fact that a child with ADD has an immaturity of the brain which means that he has less control over his behaviour. Always assess your child's behaviour and decide whether the child is *able* to change or not, given his difficulties. Your paediatrician or psychologist who carried out the diagnostic assessment will be able to guide you.

One of the great advantages of medication is that it allows children to be more successful in a behaviour modification programme because desirable behaviours increase and unwanted behaviours decrease.

You should be as consistent as possible. Decide on the limits of what your child may and may not do, and then try to stick to them. Complete consistency is, of course, impossible, but aim for as much consistency as possible. You should not be discouraged if others do not set the same limits as you do. Children with ADD can accept different limits from different people. What confuses them is when one person acts inconsistently.

Always ask yourself if some practical change would make a behaviour easier to manage. This may be simpler than embarking on a behaviour management programme. For example, behaviour management could be tried with a child with ADD who continually enters an older brother's or sister's bedroom and untidies it. However, the easiest way to resolve the problem may be to put a bolt and combination lock on the sibling's door that can be opened and locked by the sibling, but not by the child with ADD. Sometimes parents resist such an approach because they feel they do not want their home to feel like a prison. This is much better than a home which feels like a battlefield!

A child with ADD who cannot resist taking chocolate bars from the grocery cupboard because of his insatiability and poor impulse control, may be controlled by the installation of child-proof locks, or by hiding the chocolates. Sometimes parents are so close to the problem, and under so much stress, that they find it difficult to stand back and think of these practical solutions.

Many children with ADD demonstrate a number of unwanted behaviours. You will need to decide which you want to tackle first. It is usually only possible to successfully tackle one behaviour at a time. Sometimes the choice is easy; the most worrying behaviour may be the most amenable to change. Sometimes behaviours are related, and eradicating one may get rid of others. If you are feeling overwhelmed by a number of behaviour problems, it may be more rewarding to tackle a relatively minor problem first. Your quick success may then encourage you to tackle the larger problems.

Do not ignore your own stress. It is very difficult to manage a child's behaviour when you are at breaking point. Children with ADD can be extremely stressful to parents because they do not obey reasonable rules, and the behaviour of a difficult child can create tremendous stress in a family and drive parents apart. Both parents need a chance to express their feelings about the child. There are times when you need to get away and have a break. It may be a matter of having your child minded while you go for a walk, listen to some music, or soak in a warm bath.

The basis of many of the undesirable behaviours in children with ADD is poor self-esteem. Often children behave poorly at home because of negative experiences at school with their peers or a teacher. If these antecedents are understood, much can be done to decrease behaviours by building up the child's self-esteem, as discussed in chapter 10.

Some children behave less well as they become tired at the end of the day, and this may also need to be taken into consideration.

Some children may have behaviour difficulties because their medicine is not covering the entire waking period. Sometimes children's behaviour may become worse as the medicine wears off, an effect known as 'rebound'. For this reason, difficulties in a child's behaviour should always be discussed with your child's paediatrician.

In many children the onset of puberty is associated with worsening of behaviour. Although puberty is a time when the brain may mature and the ADD resolve, for some this does not happen and the only effect of puberty is the worsening of behaviour due to the effect of the hormones on the brain. Parents often do not realise that the hormonal changes associated with puberty start some two to three years before the physical changes are seen in the body. Knowing that the behaviours are due to the hormonal effects of puberty may make you feel more able to bear them. In most children, this difficult phase will usually pass when the initial rapid changes of puberty are over.

Many parents find it difficult to plan and implement a behaviour management programme on their own. If, after trying the methods described above, you have not succeeded, do not hesitate to consult your doctor and ask for a referral to a psychologist. A psychologist will spend time finding out about the child's behaviour and also about the home situation. He or she will then be able to plan, with your help, what you need to do to modify the behaviour. He or she will keep in contact with you and provide advice if further problems arise.

Summary points

- Most parents practise behaviour modification without realising it. Behaviour modification is a form of teaching employed in situations where explanation alone does not succeed.

- Always take into account the fact that a child with ADD has an immaturity of the brain which means that she has less control over her behaviour.
- One of the great advantages of medication is that it enables a behaviour modification programme to be more effective.
- Always ask yourself if some practical change would make a behaviour easier to manage. This may be simpler than embarking on a behaviour management programme.
- If you are feeling overwhelmed by a number of behaviour problems, it may be more rewarding to tackle a relatively minor problem first.
- Do not hesitate to consult your doctor and ask for a referral to a psychologist for behaviour management advice.

thirteen

Medicines—general principles

As explained in chapter 8, evidence from many sources points to low levels of neurotransmitters in the frontal part of the brain as the cause of ADD.

On the basis of this evidence, the ideal treatment for ADD would be a medicine that increased production of these neurotransmitters to levels appropriate for the child's age. Fortunately, several such medicines exist.

In every child with ADD, consideration should be given to the use of one of these medicines as part of the treatment. Ideally, such a medicine would be administered to the child from an early age, before problems with poor self-esteem, social difficulties, academic failure, and family stress have caused irreversible harm. In a child who is receiving an appropriate medicine, all other forms of treatment, such as educational and psychological intervention, will be more effective.

These medicines help the child's brain to function like the brains of other, normal children; they do not sedate the child. Most, but not all, children will be helped by medication. It is important to note that these medicines offer treatment, not a cure. This means that their effect on behaviour lasts only as long as the medicine remains in the child's body, although any skills the child has learned will persist.

How do the medicines work?

All the medicines used to treat ADD increase the amount of one or both of the neurotransmitters dopamine and norepinephrine. Each acts on one or more of the steps involved in the release, re-uptake, breakdown, and autoregulation of these neurotransmitters at the nerve ending (synapse).

Figure 6 is a schematic representation of these steps, which were described in chapter 8.

Table 5 lists the medicines used in the treatment of ADD and their site of action. Some of the medicines act at several points in the synapse, but only the most important action in ADD is listed in the table.

Precisely where each medicine acts has been discovered by research in biochemical pharmacology, the study of how med-

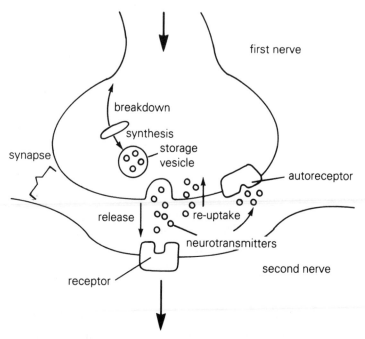

Figure 6 The pathway of neurotransmitter release, re-uptake, and breakdown at the synapse. The autoreceptor responsible for feedback is also shown.

Table 5   How medicines used in ADD increase levels of dopamine and/or norepinephrine in the synapse

Name	Major action in ADD
Methylphenidate (Ritalin)	Releases dopamine from storage vesicles
Dexamphetamine	Inhibits re-uptake of dopamine
Imipramine (Tofranil)	Inhibits re-uptake of norepinephrine
Clonidine (Catapres, Dixirit)	Blocks norepinephrine auto-receptors
Moclobemide (Aurorix)	Inhibits breakdown of dopamine and norepinephrine by monoamine oxidase
Thioridazine (Melleril)	Blocks dopamine auto-receptors

icines change the chemistry of the body. For example, because the action of methylphenidate (Ritalin) is blocked by the drug reserpine, while that of dexamphetamine is not, differences between the action of Ritalin and dexamphetamine can be studied. Reserpine depletes dopamine and norepinephrine from storage vesicles, indicating that Ritalin acts by releasing these neurotransmitters from the storage vesicles.

Some medicines used in ADD are also used for other conditions, but treatment of ADD requires smaller doses. These medicines have different effects on the neurotransmitter pathway in different doses. For example, low doses of Tofranil (imipramine) are used to treat ADD, and increase the amount of norepinephrine in the synapse by reducing its re-uptake by the nerve cell. The same medicine is used in larger doses to treat depression, where its action on the re-uptake of another neurotransmitter, serotonin, is responsible for its antidepressant effect.

The information in Table 5 suggests that a specific medicine that helps one child with ADD may not help another child, depending on which particular step in the neurotransmitter pathway is defective.

This has been found to be the case. Some children with ADD are helped by only one particular medicine. Other children are helped by a number of medicines.

These individual responses probably depend on which part of the neurotransmitter pathway is affected. For example, a child who has a defect in the release of dopamine from the storage vesicles, would be helped by methylphenidate (Ritalin), which exerts its action mainly on this step of the neurotransmitter pathway. By contrast, a child who breaks down dopamine excessively would be helped by moclobemide, which acts by inhibiting this step.

All these medicines exert their action only while they are present in the body. They do not influence the age-dependent maturational system of neurotransmitter production. They play their role by enabling the child to have normal (or near-normal) levels of neurotransmitter, until such time as his nerve cells are capable of producing adequate levels on their own.

How do we know which is the right medicine for a particular child?

The medicine for a particular child needs to be selected with care, based on a number of considerations.

First, there is the pattern of difficulties experienced by the child. Children with oppositional behaviour, for example, usually benefit from clonidine. Children with depression usually benefit from imipramine or moclobemide.

Second, there may be reasons to avoid (contraindications to) certain medicines. For example, Ritalin and dexamphetamine should be avoided in a child with ADD who has a condition known as Tourette syndrome.

After these two considerations have been taken into account, a suitable medicine is chosen and the child's response to the medicine is tested. The most thorough way of carrying this out is by means of a two-stage trial.

The two-stage medicine trial

Stage 1

This stage involves comparing the child's performance on a standardised test of concentration and memory before and after taking the medicine. This is usually carried out in the paediatrician's rooms.

This first stage of the trial is important because some children's learning deteriorates after they take a medicine that is unsuitable for them, even though their behaviour may improve. The first-stage testing also allows certain side-effects to be detected early, and can be used to determine the most appropriate dosage.

Computerised testing provides a very precise measure of performance and is often used for first-stage testing. Children enjoy this kind of test as it is similar to a computer game.

First, a standardised test is administered to the child. He then takes a dose of the medicine to be evaluated and waits for an hour until the medicine has been absorbed. A second test is then administered which is different from, but of equal difficulty to, the first.

There are many factors that can affect a child's performance over a short time period, and the results of a first-stage trial should be interpreted with care.

If the child's performance on the second test is worse than on the first, this is known as an adverse response. If an adverse response occurs, a first-stage trial with another medicine, or with a different dose of the same medicine, is usually necessary.

If there is a statistically significant improvement after the medicine, this is known as a positive response. The child should then embark on a second-stage trial with that medicine.

Stage 2

The second-stage trial of the medicine occurs in the home and/or school environment. There are many rating scales that can be used to evaluate the child's performance in these situations.

For school evaluation of medicine, it is best if the teacher monitors the child's performance without knowing when the child is on medicine.

Over a period of four weeks, the medicine is given according to a schedule known only to the doctor and parents. During this time the teacher keeps a daily record of the child's behaviour using a rating scale such as that shown in Table 4 on page 137.

At the end of the period, the parents and teacher compare the teacher's ratings with the pattern of administration of the medicine. If the medicine is helpful, the child's behaviour and learning should show significant improvement on the treatment days. With adequate explanation by the doctor, the teacher should be prepared to take part in this kind of trial.

Which aspects of ADD do the medicines help?

Few groups of medicine have been subjected to as much research as those used in ADD. The majority of the studies have focused on methylphenidate (Ritalin), but there have been many evaluations of the other medicines in the group as well.

This research has measured a number of treatment outcomes. It has involved objective measurements of children's performance, as well as the subjective ratings by parents, teachers, and peers. The studies have shown that when children with ADD take an appropriate medicine, the improvement is wide-ranging.

Table 6 lists a small sample of the many studies that have demonstrated improvement in children with ADD when taking medicine.

Learning

A large number of studies have found that medicine enhances performance on measures of vigilance, fine-motor coordination, impulsivity, and reaction time. Positive effects have also

Table 6   Some of the beneficial effects of medicine in ADD

Improved classroom learning
Balthazor, Wagner and Pelham: *Journal of Abnormal Child Psychology* 1991, vol.19: pages 35–52.

Improved academic productivity and accuracy
Douglas, Barr, O'Neill and Britton: *Journal of Child Psychology and Psychiatry* 1988, vol 29: pages 453–475.

Improved perceptual efficiency
Rappaport, DuPaul, Stoner and Jones: *Journal of Clinical Child Psychology* 1986, vol 54: pages 334–341.

Improved short-term memory
Swanson, Kinsbourne, Roberts and Zucker: *Pediatrics* 1978, vol 61: pages 21–29.

Improved vigilance, concentration, and learning
Gadow, *Children on Medication*, Volume 1, Little, Brown and Co, Boston 1986.

Improved quality of interaction with parents
Barkley, Karlsson, Strzelecki and Murphy: *Journal of Consulting and Clinical Psychology* 1984, vol 52: pages 750–758.

Improved response to a behaviour modification programme
Gittelman, Abikoff, Pollack, Klein, Katz and Mattes in: *Hyperactive Children: The Social Ecology of Identification and Treatment* Academic Press, New York 1980.

Improved quality of interaction with teachers and peers
Pelham, Bender Caddell, Booth and Moore: *Archives of General Psychiatry* 1985, vol 42: pages 948–952.

Less restless and more 'normal' in class
Barkley and Cunningham: *American Journal of Orthopsychiatry* 1979, vol 49: pages 491–499.

Less aggressive
Gadow, Nolan, Sverd, Sprafkin, and Paolicelli: *Journal of the American Academy of Child and Adolescent Psychiatry* 1990, vol 29: pages 710–718.

Less negative and disruptive in the classroom and playground
Pelham, Bender Caddell, Booth and Moore: *Archives of General Psychiatry* 1985, vol 42: pages 948–952.

Improved standing among classmates and greater social acceptance
Whalen, Henker and Dotemoto: *Child Development* 1981, vol 58: pages 816–828.

Table 6   Some of the beneficial effects of medicine in ADD *(continued)*

More likely to be rated as 'best friend' or 'fun' by peers
Whalen, Henker, Buhrmester, Hinshaw, Huber and Laski: *Journal of Consulting and Clinical Psychology* 1989, vol 57: pages 545–549.

Better sporting performance
Pelham, McBurnett, Harper, Milich, Murphy, Clinton and Thiele: *Journal of Consulting and Clinical Psychology* 1990, vol 58: pages 130–133.

---

been obtained on measures of learning and memory, both for non-verbal and verbal material.

Studies have shown that children become better at simple and complex learning procedures. They are better able to remember words and symbols they have learned. They can recall information they have learned more rapidly and more accurately.

None of the learning that occurs in children on medicine is 'state dependent'. This means that skills and knowledge acquired while a child is on medicine do not wear off when the medicine is no longer taken.

Recent studies have also shown that medicine can improve academic productivity and accuracy in children with ADD. Handwriting becomes neater and task persistence improves.

Behaviour

Medicine also results in dramatic effects on behaviour. There is improvement in concentration on assigned tasks. Children on medicine are more settled and less over-active. They become less impulsive and disruptive. They become more compliant. Aggression is markedly reduced.

A common fear is that the use of medicine will make the child overly compliant and take away her natural exuberance and sparkle. This is not the case. While children with ADD do become better able to conform to reasonable rules when taking medicine, they nevertheless remain slightly more active and impulsive than their peers. Medicine certainly does not transform them into anergic automatons.

Social skills

Medicine also helps children with their social interactions. Negative behaviours are reduced and children become less defiant. Interactions with peers improve greatly. Children are less likely to behave in a 'silly', immature, and over-excited manner. In one study, peers consistently rated children with ADD as being more 'fun' when they were on their medicine. This observation was made without the peers knowing when the children with ADD were on their medicine.

Emotional state

The medicines also have an effect on children's mood. Children generally become more positive about themselves and more confident in day-to-day activities. Parents report that their children become more reasonable and that outbursts of anger decrease in frequency and intensity.

Many parents have observed that their child became more outgoing and more communicative on medication.

The place of medicine in the treatment of ADD

Medicine has the potential to reduce many of the difficulties experienced by children with ADD. In many children, the change is dramatic. It is not unusual for the change in the child to be described as miraculous. Often the child seems to be completely transformed when on treatment. This is because the child is able to behave in a more mature, age-appropriate manner.

For some children, medicine may so improve their competence that no other form of special treatment is needed. Ordinary educational programmes and average parental rearing practices are sufficient for their needs. For other children, medicine alone is not enough and must be used in conjunction with individualised educational and behaviour management programmes.

Not every child will respond to these medicines; some 10 per cent of children are not helped by any of the medicines currently available.

The decision about whether a child should take medication should be made by the parents on the advice of their child's paediatrician. This should follow a comprehensive assessment, as outlined in chapter 9. Whenever possible, the child should be involved in the decision as well.

Can children with ADD be treated adequately without medication?

Some children with mild ADD can manage to overcome their difficulties with non-medical intervention. However, for children with moderate or severe ADD, behaviour management and educational strategies are inadequate when used alone. Why is this the case?

Behaviour modification is based on rewarding desirable behaviour and ignoring undesirable behaviour. This is often impractical in children with ADD, because desirable behaviour is too infrequently displayed to allow reinforcement. Undesirable behaviour, on the other hand, may be so disruptive or dangerous that it cannot be ignored.

The memory and attention of many children with ADD are so impaired that they do not benefit adequately from educational programmes, without the help of medication.

Another problem with non-medical treatments for ADD is that, in situations where parents and teachers are not able to be present, the child may fail miserably.

For example, in his social interactions (when adults cannot play a role) the child with ADD may have a great deal of trouble because of his poor social cognition. This is often compounded by peers responding in a way that is detrimental to the child.

When he needs to occupy himself, or organise his work independently, the child with ADD often becomes dysfunctional because he lacks the necessary self-direction and self-organisation skills.

In these situations, the child with ADD may enter a vicious cycle. He fails because of his difficulties and then does not want to try again because he fears further failure.

Medication offers the child with ADD the opportunity to escape this vicious cycle and enter what might be called a 'virtuous cycle'. Because the child becomes more competent when taking the medicine, other forms of treatment, such as behaviour modification and education programmes, become more effective. With the medicine playing its role, there is a reduction in undesirable behaviour. The child can therefore receive more appropriate praise. He also becomes more attentive during class and remedial work and his learning improves.

As the child becomes more successful, both at home and in school, he is prepared to attempt new tasks and to face new challenges. As he succeeds in these, his learning and behaviour improve. It is not surprising, therefore, that children with ADD often surge ahead once on medicine.

Studies such as those of Rachel Gittelmann and her associates have demonstrated that the best results are obtained by combining medicine with other strategies: the 'multi-modal' approach.

Explaining the role of medicine to your child

For the best results, it is essential that your child understands the role of the medicine.

First, emphasise to your child that she *is* able to concentrate, but that this requires a great deal of effort on her part. It is essential that she realises that she does have the ability to concentrate, and that she does not feel that the medicine will be used because she is unable to do this at all. Explain that the role of the medicine is to make it easier for her to concentrate.

The analogy of wearing glasses (spectacles) is useful. Explain that in the same way some children wear glasses to make seeing easier, some children need medicine to make concentrating easier. Emphasise that in the same way that glasses do not dictate what the wearer should look at, so the medicine will not control what she concentrates on. She will still have to decide what she wants to concentrate on; the medicine will allow her to do this more effectively, with greater ease, and for longer periods of time.

Explain also that when one puts on a pair of glasses, one does not instantly acquire knowledge. Similarly, the tablets contain no knowledge, they will only help her to learn more effectively. She will still need to complete her work and to commit it to memory. The medicine is only an aid.

A child with ADD embarking on treatment with medicine needs to know that her progress will be carefully monitored and that she will be given a guide as to how she is progressing. She also needs to know that the time will come when she will no longer require the medicine and that she can then stop taking it.

Most children are only too happy to have this kind of help. Some may, however, not want other children to know that they are taking medicine. Peers may say inappropriate things, and children with ADD do not want to be teased about having to take tablets to help them. The dose that usually gives problems in this regard is the one that is taken during school hours. This should be taken in private. For the older, more competent child, it is best if the tablet is packed with her lunch, so that she can take it during her break. The tablet can be hidden in a marshmallow, or chocolate, so that it can be swallowed without anyone else being aware. Some children take an extra plain marshmallow of a different colour in case they are asked for one by a friend. These forms of harmless subterfuge are necessary to ensure that children take their medicine without drawing attention to themselves.

It is essential that all concerned, parents, teachers, and siblings, do not say things such as, 'You are behaving badly—go and take your medicine!' The taking of medicine should be a routine event, like brushing teeth; it should not attract comment.

With the intensive anti-drug campaigns directed towards children, it is not surprising that many are against the idea of regular medication. Explain that there is a great difference between a 'street drug' and a medicine prescribed by a doctor. It is not drug abuse to take a medicine prescribed for a condition by a specialist who has made a specific diagnosis and who will monitor the child's progress.

Do not have unrealistic expectations of medicine

Approximately 90 per cent of children with ADD are helped by medicine. The proportion of children who are helped is greater for those with the hyperactive form of ADD than those with the dreamy, vague form of the condition. In the latter group the success rate is approximately 50 per cent.

In many children, the response to medicine is dramatic. Individuals who do not know the child is on medicine comment on how much better the child has become. If the child misses a tablet, teachers and relatives notice.

In other children, the effect is not so dramatic. Things do become easier for the child, but residual difficulties remain. In these children, medicine plays an important role, but is not the total answer to the child's difficulties.

Lastly, there is a group of children for whom medicine has no role, either because it does not help them at all, or because it actually has an adverse effect upon them. For these children, only non-medical methods of help are possible.

Medication does not cure ADD. Nevertheless, if used appropriately as part of an overall management strategy, it plays a pivotal role in preventing irreversible difficulties in self-esteem and social and academic failure.

For those individuals whose difficulties persist into adulthood, medicine can continue to play a role in helping them to achieve their potential in their work, as well as in their social and family lives (see chapter 15).

Summary points

- In every child with ADD, consideration should be given to the use of medicine as part of the treatment.

- All the medicines used to treat ADD increase the amount of the neurotransmitters dopamine and/or norepinephrine.
- Some children with ADD are helped by only one particular medicine. Some do best with a combination of medicines.
- Choice of the best medicine for a particular child is based on the pattern of difficulties in the child, the presence of any contraindications, and the results of a two-stage medicine trial.
- Medicine is able to reduce many of the difficulties experienced by children with ADD. In a great number of children, the changes caused by medicine are dramatic.
- The learning that occurs in a child on medicine is not state dependent, i.e. it does not disappear when the medicine is no longer taken.
- Medicine enables the child to be more competent so that other forms of treatment, such as behaviour modification and education programmes, become more effective.
- For some children, medicine may so improve their competence that no other form of special treatment is needed. For other children, medicine must be used in conjunction with individualised educational and behaviour management programmes.
- For the best results, it is essential that the child understands the role of medicine in helping him.
- Children should be able to take their medicine in private if they wish.
- Approximately 90 per cent of children with ADD will be helped by medicine. The proportion of children who are helped is greater for those with the hyperactive form of ADD.

fourteen

A guide to specific medicines

The medicines used in ADD are a heterogeneous group. Their main common attribute is that they all increase neurotransmitter levels at the synapse.

Some of these medicines are used almost exclusively for treating ADD. Others are also used for disorders as diverse as bedwetting, high blood pressure, migraines, and depression. They are generally prescribed in smaller doses for ADD than for these other disorders.

The vast majority of children with ADD are effectively treated with a single medicine. This is usually Ritalin (methylphenidate) or dexamphetamine. Other children need a combination of two or more medicines. The usual combinations are Ritalin and clonidine (Catapres) or dexamphetamine and clonidine.

Ritalin and dexamphetamine are short-acting medicines that do not accumulate in the body. The other medicines used in ADD act for longer and are administered in such a way as to produce a steady level in the blood stream.

This chapter deals with the main medicines used in ADD. Ritalin and dexamphetamine are described in the greatest detail because they are most commonly used.

Ritalin (Methylphenidate) and Dexamphetamine

Ritalin and dexamphetamine are related to one another; both belong to a group of medicines known as 'stimulants'. They have similar methods of action, and similar side-effects.

In a normal child, Ritalin and dexamphetamine increase neurotransmitter levels above normal, resulting in over-stimulation and over-activity. In a child with ADD, however, they have the paradoxical effect of making the child less restless and more focused. This is presumably because neurotransmitter levels are only increased to normal, or near normal, levels.

Although Ritalin and dexamphetamine are related, they have different effects on the neurotransmitter pathway. It is for this reason that some children respond better to one than to the other. This is the reason why medicine testing, described in the previous chapter, is so important.

Dexamphetamine was first used for children with ADD in 1937, when Dr Charles Bradley serendipitously discovered that it helped children who had difficulties with sustained concentration. Ritalin has been used for the same purpose since 1957.

Tablet strength

Each medicine is available in only one strength. Ritalin is manufactured as a 10 mg tablet and dexamphetamine as a 5 mg tablet. The two tablets are of equal strength or potency.

Cost

In Australia, there is presently a price difference to the consumer between Ritalin and dexamphetamine. This is because the Commonwealth Government subsidises dexamphetamine (Pharmaceutical Benefits Scheme), but not Ritalin. It is possible that Ritalin may be placed on the Pharmaceutical Benefits Scheme in the near future. The government will be reviewing this in 1995.

One hundred tablets (approximately one month's supply) of dexamphetamine cost approximately $16.00. The same number of Ritalin tablets costs approximately $70.00. If the child has a Health Care Card, the price of the dexamphetamine drops to approximately $2.50. The only way parents can obtain relief for the expense of Ritalin is through private health fund insurance. Parents of a child with ADD can apply for the Child Disability Allowance (CDA) from the Commonwealth Department of Social Security. If successful, this allowance can be used towards the cost of the child's medicine.

The price difference means many children are tried on dexamphetamine first. However, there are some children who are not helped by dexamphetamine, or may even be adversely affected by it. For some of these children, Ritalin is the only effective medicine.

Duration of action

Both Ritalin and dexamphetamine are short-acting medicines. They take effect one hour after administration and their action lasts for approximately four hours.

In some children the effect lasts for only three hours, while in others it continues for six hours. This depends on the rapidity with which the child's body metabolises or breaks down the medicine, and also on how quickly the neurotransmitter levels, once raised by the medicine, are broken down in the brain.

Dosage and administration

Both of these medicines are well absorbed with food, and it is better for children to take them after food whenever possible. Pharmacists sometimes place a note on the pack saying that the tablets should be swallowed 20 to 30 minutes before meals. This instruction should be ignored, unless confirmed by your child's doctor, because both these medicines can suppress the child's appetite.

It is best if the child takes the smallest dose required to achieve a satisfactory improvement. Some children are very sensitive to these medicines and require only a half or quarter tablet for each dose. Other children, of exactly the same size, require one and a half or two tablets for each dose.

The appropriate dose does not depend on the child's weight and age alone. It is determined by the type of difficulties the child has, his temperament, his constitution, and the speed with which he breaks down the medicine. For example, a child who is dreamy and vague needs a relatively small dose to help his concentration and working memory. If such a child is given a larger dose, his performance may deteriorate. Children who are overactive or aggressive usually need larger doses. Children who are delicate and anxious tolerate only small doses; robust children generally respond best to higher doses. The choice of the best dose to suit a child is as much an art as a science, and requires the prescribing doctor to have a great deal of experience in treating children with ADD.

In all cases, it is best to start with a small dose and to then slowly increase the dose after five or six days; this enables the child to adjust gradually to the effects of the medicine.

These are not medicines that accumulate in the body, and every child will have periods during the day, as well as during the entire night, when the medicine is absent from the body. When the medicine needs to be stopped, there is no need to withdraw it slowly; the child can abruptly stop taking it.

The first dose of the day should be given at or after breakfast, because these medicines tend to decrease appetite when they are present in the body. By waiting until after breakfast, the child will not lose her appetite for this important meal.

It is usually necessary to give a second tablet some three hours after the first.

Although the medicine acts for approximately four hours, it should be remembered that the second tablet takes about an hour to work. This is why it is given three hours after the first.

For most children, the first tablet is given after breakfast, at approximately 7.30 a.m., and the second tablet is given at recess (little lunch), at approximately 11.00 a.m. This second tablet starts working at approximately 12.00 noon, which is when the first dose of the day has worn off.

Many children require a third dose to help with the afternoon period at home. This is important in helping the child with her homework, and also with her behaviour at home. It is best if this dose is given at approximately 3.30 p.m. when the child arrives home. It should not be given later than 4.00 p.m. or it may interfere with the child's ability to fall asleep at night. Ritalin and dexamphetamine make children more alert, and this may cause insomnia.

It is often best to give a smaller amount of medicine for the third dose than for the earlier doses of the day. This has the advantage of making it easier for the child to fall asleep in the evening, and also prevents a phenomenon known as 'rebound', which may occur when the medicine abruptly wears off. 'Rebound' manifests itself by the child becoming restless or moody for a short time as the medicine suddenly stops working. By giving a half dosage for the last part of the day, the effect of the medicine subsides more gradually, and so rebound does not occur.

Some children have trouble falling asleep if they are given more than two doses per day. Children on only two doses per day should take the first at approximately 8.00 a.m. and the second at approximately 12.00 noon. With this timing there is better coverage throughout the day.

An occasional child metabolises the medicine extremely quickly and needs four or even five doses spread out through the day.

Side-effects

Both Ritalin and dexamphetamine are very well researched medicines. In fact, Ritalin is arguably the best studied of all medicines used in paediatrics.

During the time that each tablet is present in the body, appetite may decrease. To overcome this side effect, the first tablet of the day is usually given with or after breakfast. Most children on either of these medicines usually eat slightly less during the day (a time when many school children do not eat much in any case). Most children compensate for this by eating more at the end of the day, when the effect of the medicine has worn off.

When treatment with these medicines is commenced there is often a slight loss of weight over the first couple of months. In the vast majority of children, weight stabilises and then starts increasing again.

For many children with ADD who are overweight, this slight drop in weight is beneficial for their self-image. It is extremely rare for loss of weight to necessitate the withdrawal of medicine. Occasionally a reduction in dose may be necessary because of weight loss.

The second common side-effect is difficulty falling asleep at night. This is most prominent when treatment is first started, but usually resolves after one or two weeks. If insomnia persists, the last dose of the day may be reduced or omitted. Some children are very sensitive to this effect and can only tolerate a morning dose.

Other side-effects are extremely uncommon. An occasional child may suffer from headaches or abdominal discomfort when treatment is commenced. These side-effects usually disappear after a few days.

Some children become tearful, or over-subdued, on these medicines. These responses suggest that the dose of medicine is too high for the child and should be reduced. Some children will need to have the dosage reduced by half a tablet or less. The tablets are scored down the middle, but can be broken into quarters, or even eighths, with a pill cutter or sharp knife. Parents should experiment with slight modifications to the dose in order to achieve the best result. They should not hesitate to contact their child's doctor if the dose does not seem to be appropriate.

At one stage it was thought that children with epilepsy should not be given these medicines. It is now realised that seizures are rarely induced or aggravated by Ritalin or dexamphetamine.

Children who have a tendency to motor tics (involuntary twitches of parts of the body, such as the eyelids, or the head) may have their tics worsened by these medicines. This is not always the case, and some children's tics are unaffected, or may even improve. Nevertheless, a child with tics should be carefully monitored when taking Ritalin or dexamphetamine, and these medicines should be stopped if tics worsen. Other medicines for ADD can then be used, such as clonidine, which has the advantage of reducing tics.

Studies in the 1970s raised the possibility of growth suppression by Ritalin and dexamphetamine. Later studies have shown that this is a dose-related phenomenon, probably related to a decrease in appetite. It is a transient effect that occurs primarily in the first year of treatment, and seems to have no effect on eventual adult height. Nevertheless, growth of children receiving these medicines should be monitored regularly by their paediatrician.

Parents are sometimes concerned because both of these medicines are potentially addictive. It must be emphasised that there is no risk of a child with ADD becoming addicted to either of these medicines when they are used properly. Addiction only occurs when large amounts of the medicine are taken by adults who aim to escape reality. Children with ADD are treated with small amounts of medicine to help them focus on the reality around them. Long-term studies have shown that there is no increase in the rate of addiction in children with ADD who are treated with these medicines. When these medicines are no longer required, there is no need for a withdrawal period; the child simply stops taking them.

Some children might become overactive, irritable, or tearful at the time that the effects of a tablet wear off. This short-lasting phenomenon is known as 'rebound'. Some children will cope with this by becoming involved in a physical activity. Parents who realise that their child is having this reaction for a short period of time may encourage him to go outside and play, or to sit quietly and watch television. During such periods, it is important not to make excessive demands on the child. Often a half dosage of the medicine given on return from school abolishes afternoon rebound.

Should Ritalin and dexamphetamine be taken on weekends?

Children whose only difficulty relates to schoolwork, need take their medicine on school days only.

An occasional child with school-based difficulties may find that he has problems falling asleep on Monday nights, because his body has to adjust to the re-introduction of the medicine after each weekend break. In such a case, it may be better for the child to take the medicine seven days a week.

Children who have difficulties at home and at school should be given the benefit of medicine seven days a week. For such children, their condition, and the difficulties they face, are present seven days a week and there is no reason to withhold medicine on weekends. Taking the medicine seven days a week allows such children's behaviour to be far more consistent, and consequently they have greater opportunities to learn and succeed throughout the week. It is not fair to such children to deprive them of their treatment on weekends.

For most children who take medicine on weekends, the dosage regime can be more flexible on Saturdays and Sundays than on other days of the week. For example, a child who takes medicine at 7.30 a.m., 11.00 a.m., and 3.30 p.m. on weekdays may find it easier to take the medicine after a late breakfast and after lunch (2 doses only) on Saturdays and Sundays.

If a child plays sport on weekends, the medicine might be given one hour before a game. This allows the child to be more focused during the game, and therefore more successful.

A child who has remedial lessons on weekends can also time his dose so that he takes a tablet one hour before the lesson. This will enable him to concentrate and persist with tasks more effectively during the lessons.

During school holidays, a child who has difficulties with behaviour should be kept on his medicine unless there is a special reason to stop it, such as the need to gain weight.

When to stop treatment

The decision about ceasing the medicine should be reviewed every six months. Many children will continue to need their treatment until they reach the age of 16 or 18 years. This means that many children will need to take the medicine for several years. The safety of these medicines when used in this way is well established.

Long-acting formulations

Both Ritalin and dexamphetamine are available in the United States of America in long-acting forms. These are Ritalin SR (Sustained Release), a 20 mg tablet, and 'Dexedrine (dexamphetamine) Spansules', available as 5 mg, 10 mg, and 15 mg capsules. None of these preparations is available in Australia.

Although the idea of a longer duration of action sounds attractive, these formulations produce unreliable blood levels, take longer to work, and are generally less effective in controlling symptoms than the short-acting forms.

In the USA, another closely related stimulant, pemoline (Cylert), is also available. It can be obtained in Australia with the special consent of the Commonwealth Department of Health. Pemoline should be avoided because it carries a risk of causing liver damage.

Tofranil (Imipramine)

Tofranil has been used for many years to treat bedwetting in children, as well as to treat depression in both children and adults. Over the last decade its usefulness in children with ADD has been well established.

It is used in smaller doses in children with ADD than for bedwetting and depression. However, in children with ADD who have bedwetting or depression in addition to ADD, larger doses can be taken.

Tofranil is a long-acting medicine that remains in the body for some eight hours after a tablet is taken. The medicine is given regularly with the aim of achieving a steady level in the blood. For this reason, the exact timing of each dose is not as critical as it is for Ritalin and dexamphetamine.

Because the blood level must be built up slowly, it usually takes two weeks before the full action of Tofranil becomes evident.

Tofranil will help with all the major difficulties seen in children with ADD. It improves concentration, decreases impulsivity, and reduces oppositional behaviour.

Dosage and administration

The aim of treatment with Tofranil is to achieve a steady level in the blood and consequently the medicine is given seven days a week. The first tablet is given with breakfast, the second can be given at lunchtime, or on return from school. Sometimes a third tablet is given in the evening as well. The medicine is available in two sizes: 10 mg and 25 mg tablets.

Side-effects

Tofranil is used in such low doses for ADD that side-effects are uncommon. When treatment is first started, the child may suffer from sleepiness or easy fatigability, but these are usually mild and resolve after a week or two.

Other possible side-effects are slight dryness of the mouth (which can be helpful in children who tend to dribble), constipation, and excessive perspiration. It is very rare for these side-effects to be troublesome enough to necessitate stopping the medicine. Constipation can usually be counteracted by ensuring that the child has sufficient dietary fibre.

The occasional child will have a decrease in appetite on Tofranil, but this is rarely as prominent as with Ritalin or dexamphetamine.

One of the drawbacks of Tofranil is that the positive effects may wear off over time. This is known as the development of 'tolerance', and may be remedied by raising the dose, or stopping the medicine for a period before re-introducing it.

Withdrawal

When the Tofranil is no longer needed, it is usual to withdraw it gradually over a couple of weeks so as to prevent 'rebound depression'. This is not necessary if the dose taken is less than 20 mg a day.

Clonidine (Catapres, Dixirit)

In the late 1970s it was first proposed that clonidine, a medicine that had been used for a decade to treat migraine and high blood pressure, might be effective in treating ADD. This has now been well established.

The main effect of clonidine is on the neurotransmitter norepinephrine and it is extremely effective in children with oppositional or aggressive behaviour.

Clonidine combines very well with either Ritalin or dexamphetamine, and children can be treated with combinations of clonidine and one of these two medicines. Often the effect of clonidine in combination with these medicines results in better control of the ADD, as well as a reduction in side-effects. This is because clonidine counteracts one of the main side-effects of Ritalin and dexamphetamine: insomnia. Clonidine promotes sleep and so it often cures the insomnia caused by Ritalin or dexamphetamine.

Clonidine has a greater effect on behaviour, particularly aggression, temper tantrums, and defiance, than it does on concentration. For this reason the combination with Ritalin or dexamphetamine (both of whose primary action is on concentration) is complementary.

Clonidine, like Tofranil, is a long-acting medicine and must be given regularly in order to achieve a constant level in the bloodstream. It is given at least twice a day, and in some children up to four times a day, in order to achieve a steady level in the blood. Clonidine must be taken seven days a week.

When treatment is commenced, the improvement may not be evident for several weeks. The earliest effect is usually observed after ten days, but it may take two or three months before the maximal beneficial effect is apparent.

Dosage and administration

Clonidine is available in a small, coated tablet (Dixirit, 25 microgram) marketed to prevent migraine, and a larger uncoated, white tablet (Catapres, 100 microgram) used to treat high blood pressure. Either of these preparations can be used, but Catapres tablets will need to be broken into quarters or halves for most children with ADD.

Catapres is cheaper than Dixirit, as it is on the Pharmaceutical Benefits Scheme. Some parents may be prepared to pay the extra for the convenience of the sugar-coated Dixirit formulation, which does not have to be broken and is therefore easier for children to take to school.

In the USA, clonidine is also available in the form of a skin patch, which is a small bandage impregnated with the medicine that adheres to the skin (usually on the back). The medicine is then absorbed steadily through the skin during the day. This avoids the necessity for repeated tablet taking. The only danger is that the child may pull off the skin patch. Skin patches are more expensive than tablets and are presently unavailable in Australia.

Side-effects

Clonidine is free of any significant side-effects when used in the doses usually required for ADD. Some children may become drowsy when they first start this medicine, but this side-effect quickly subsides.

Clonidine is usually used in such small doses in ADD that there is no appreciable effect on blood pressure. Some children may feel dizzy if the dose is excessive, and this may indicate that their blood pressure is being lowered. The dose should then be reduced.

Parents should be aware that behaviour *may initially deteriorate* when treatment with clonidine commences. If treatment is continued, the positive effects will be seen after two or three weeks. Parents may therefore have to prepare for some worsening of behaviour when treatment with clonidine is started.

For children who have migraines in addition to ADD, treatment with clonidine may prevent their headaches, as clonidine is also used in small doses to treat migraine. Ironically, despite its use to treat migraine, clonidine can *cause* headaches in some children.

Withdrawal

When treatment involves the use of more than 50 micrograms of clonidine a day, the medicine should be withdrawn slowly over a period of two to three weeks to prevent 'rebound hypertension', a condition where blood pressure rises on sudden cessation of clonidine. When a child is taking a dose above 50 micrograms a day, he should not miss a dose for the same reason. However, even if a dose is missed, it is extremely unlikely that any harm will ensue.

If treatment involves less than 50 micrograms per day, clonidine can be stopped abruptly when no longer needed.

Aurorix (Moclobemide)

The destruction of the neurotransmitters dopamine and norepinephrine in nerve cells involves an enzyme known as a monoamine oxidase. The action of this enzyme can be counteracted by medicines known as monoamine oxidase inhibitors (MAO-I). Their effect is to increase the amount of these neurotransmitters in the synapse.

MOA inhibitors have been used for a long time to treat depression. However, they have always had the disadvantage that people taking such a medicine had to be careful not to eat certain foods (such as cheese) because of the risk of dangerous interactions. This made the use of MOA inhibitors in children with ADD fraught with difficulties.

Now a second generation of MOA inhibitors has been developed that are reversible, and do not require any dietary restrictions. One of these, Aurorix (moclobemide), is very effective in treating some children with ADD.

Dose and administration

Aurorix is usually given in a dose of 75 mg twice a day (i.e. half a tablet twice a day). Increasing the dose does not result in a better response. However, the dose may be increased if a child has depression in association with ADD, so that the Aurorix can treat the depression as well.

The medicine is given seven days a week, and it usually takes one or two weeks before the effect is apparent. When the medicine is no longer needed, it is best to withdraw it slowly.

The child can remain on her usual diet while taking this medicine.

Side-effects

Aurorix is very free of side-effects. Difficulties with falling asleep and a decrease in appetite may occur, but are rare.

Melleril (Thioridazine)

Melleril can be a very effective medicine in children with ADD. It is used mainly for children in whom oppositional or aggressive behaviour is a major problem. However, it may help behaviour and at the same time have an adverse effect on learning, so all children taking this medicine for ADD should have their academic attainments carefully monitored.

Melleril is a long-acting medicine and must be given two or three times a day on a regular basis to achieve a therapeutic response. It should be given seven days a week. It usually takes two weeks before the full effect is seen.

Side-effects

Melleril may cause sleepiness but this usually subsides after a few days.

It may increase appetite, which can be a problem in children who are obese.

Melleril increases the sensitivity of the skin to sunburn, so sunscreens should be used when the child is exposed to the sun.

A particular concern with high doses of Melleril for extended periods is the possibility of developing muscular stiffness and abnormal movements. Very occasionally, these abnormal movements may persist even when the medicine is ceased. These side-effects mean that Melleril should only be used if no other medicine for ADD is suitable. Melleril should always be given in the smallest effective dose and should not be continued for longer than is necessary.

Despite these concerns, Melleril can play a very important role in helping some children with ADD when no other medicine is effective. Used conservatively and with proper monitoring, this medicine can be taken for several years with no adverse effects.

Other medicines

Many of the medicines used in ADD were first developed for other conditions before their effectiveness in ADD was noted. It is anticipated that many medicines currently used for conditions such as depression and anxiety may be found to be effective in children with ADD.

Already medicines such as fluoxetine (Prozac), an antidepressant, and propranolol (Inderal), a medicine used to prevent anxiety symptoms, have been found to be effective in some children with ADD. It is to be expected that the list of medicines used for children with ADD will lengthen over the next decade.

Summary points

- The vast majority of children with ADD are effectively treated with a single medicine. This is usually Ritalin or dexamphetamine.
- There is a widespread misconception that children with ADD are given medicines that sedate them. The truth is that most children with ADD are given stimulants.

- Although Ritalin and dexamphetamine are related, they have different actions. It is for this reason that some children with ADD respond better to the one than to the other.
- It is best if the child takes the smallest effective dose of a medicine.
- All medicines can have side-effects, but the safety and efficacy of medicines used in ADD are well established.
- Clonidine is effective in children with oppositional and aggressive behaviour. It works well in combination with Ritalin or dexamphetamine.
- Children with tics may be better treated with clonidine, or Tofranil, than Ritalin or dexamphetamine.

Adulthood

fifteen

Will the child grow out of it?

A decade ago the general consensus was that children with ADD would invariably grow out of their problems. This has now been disproved. In a sizeable proportion of children with ADD, the difficulties persist into adulthood. Such difficulties may take the form of residual ADD, secondary problems, or a combination of the two.

Residual ADD

When the difficulties associated with ADD, such as poor attention span, impulsivity, and restlessness, persist into adult life, this is known as 'residual ADD' (rADD).

In the vast majority of children with ADD, these difficulties decrease during late adolescence. This may be a gradual decrease between the ages of 12 and 18 years, or may occur more abruptly (usually around 16–18 years). In some children the improvement in the late teenage years is so marked that their ADD can be regarded as having completely resolved. This probably occurs in some 20 per cent of children with ADD.

In approximately 80 per cent of children with ADD, the improvement in the teenage years will not be associated with a complete resolution, and 60 per cent will have mild residual ADD and 20 per cent a severe form.

Adults with *mild* residual ADD will usually not be hampered by their condition. Many will simply 'bypass' their difficulties by making career and other life choices so that their difficulties with sustained attention, social cognition or impulsivity do not interfere with their day-to-day functioning.

Some adults with this residual form of ADD may even turn some of their 'difficulties' into advantages. For example, a certain degree of restlessness may help such a person attain goals, because it makes him more energetic and less prone to become tired than other people. Impulsivity of thought can also be turned into an advantage if it allows the individual to think laterally and innovatively. Even some minor difficulties with social cognition may allow the individual to be more successful in some endeavours where being forthright is an advantage. Many individuals with mild residual ADD do extremely well in the business world.

In approximately 20 per cent of children with ADD, difficulties persist into adulthood in a *severe* form. These individuals have residual ADD which often hampers their family life and their work. It is these individuals for whom on-going treatment of ADD during adulthood is essential. This will be discussed later in the chapter.

Secondary problems

The term 'residual ADD' refers to persistence of the characteristics of ADD, such as impulsivity and restlessness, into adulthood. Many adults who had ADD during childhood will have other, secondary problems that arose *because* of their ADD in childhood.

For example, their ADD may have resulted in their inability to achieve good academic skills, or may have undermined their self-esteem.

Whether or not the ADD itself persists, many adults who had ADD in childhood will continue to suffer as a result of these complications.

At the present moment, we have no way of preventing residual ADD. The continued difficulties of ADD are presumably related to genetic problems that are beyond our control. However, by early treatment of children with ADD, we can certainly avoid or diminish the secondary problems that ADD causes during childhood and which may then persist into adult life.

It is important to distinguish secondary problems from residual problems. Secondary problems may exist in adults who have residual ADD, as well as in adults in whom the primary characteristics of ADD have resolved. The latter group may still need help in the form of counselling, adult education, self-support groups, and specialist help with career advice and employment support. A person with secondary problems who does *not* have residual ADD would not benefit from medication. This is quite different from adults with residual ADD, where medication may play a very important role in helping ameliorate the symptoms of ADD.

Characteristics of residual ADD

Residual ADD is due to the persistence of the features of childhood ADD described in chapter 1. The characteristics are very similar, but with adulthood the nature of some problems changes.

Adults with ADD have tremendous difficulty completing projects. They will often have a number of different projects that they are tackling simultaneously without properly following through any of them. Their difficulties with task persistence often involve procrastination; they have great difficulty getting started with a task.

Easy distractability and difficulties focusing attention are common. Many adults with ADD complain that they tend to lose track when reading. Their partners and children often complain that they 'tune out' when they speak to them.

Impatience is a very prominent characteristic in residual ADD. Adults with ADD are very intolerant of 'red tape'. They have difficulty going through necessary procedures and often develop reputations for being mavericks.

They are very restless individuals and are intolerant of what they regard as 'boring' activities. They find it very difficult to relax in leisure activities that do not require a high level of activity. They have a low tolerance for frustration and quickly lose their temper or give up if a task requires persistence. They have particular difficulty working at tedious tasks that require incentival motivation (motivation for a reward that is far off in the future).

Adults with ADD find it difficult to get themselves organised. They can be very creative and intuitive, but will often need someone else to ensure that the more practical, day-to-day arrangements are made.

Impulsivity is a particular problem for adults with residual ADD. For many, it is the most prominent characteristic. Impulsivity may be seen verbally, in a tendency to say what comes into their mind without necessarily considering the timing or appropriateness of the remark. This may create difficulties in personal and professional interactions. Impulsivity may also be seen in a tendency to spend money, change plans, and enact new schemes at very short notice. These difficulties may not be apparent to the person with ADD himself, but may cause great problems to family and co-workers.

Many adults with ADD suffer because of poor memory. Many come to rely on aids such as writing everything down and placing reminders all over their homes and workplaces.

Another common area of difficulty is in self-appraisal. Adults with ADD are often very inaccurate in their self-observation. They may have little idea of the impact that they are having on other people. This does not mean that they lack concern. They often have a tendency to worry needlessly about things. Many complain about a sense of impending doom or insecurity. Mood swings are also common.

The problems with self-esteem described in chapter 7 may persist into adulthood. Some degree of depression is therefore common in adults with residual ADD.

In some adults with residual ADD, risk-taking behaviour is a problem. Such individuals search for high stimulation. In some cases this may be found in activities such as sport or public life. Occasionally a tendency is shown towards addictive behaviour, such as substance abuse, or activities such as gambling.

It can be seen that adults with ADD are 'high risk' individuals. Many of their attributes may cause them to be extremely successful and to become 'high flyers'. However, they are also in danger of experiencing problems in personal relationships and with their financial affairs.

How is the diagnosis of residual ADD made?

Many of the characteristics of residual ADD are seen in normal adults. Everyone can be, to some extent, distractable, restless, and impulsive. The diagnosis of residual ADD depends upon the duration and intensity of these problems, as well as the characteristic clustering of features.

The diagnosis may then be confirmed by psychometric and neuro-electrophysiological testing similar to that carried out in children with suspected ADD.

ADD always starts in childhood. It is therefore a prerequisite for the diagnosis that the characteristics have been present throughout the person's life. In some cases, the diagnosis of ADD will already have been made during childhood, but sometimes the diagnosis is first made in adulthood.

If it is clear that a child with ADD will continue to have problems during adulthood, the paediatrician who looks after him will refer him to a psychiatrist once the child reaches the age of 18 years. An adult who thinks he may have ADD should request that his general practitioner refer him to a psychiatrist for an assessment.

Certain psychiatrists have a particular interest in residual ADD and therefore have experience and expertise in this area. They may work in conjunction with psychologists who carry out standardised testing to evaluate the individual's particular strengths and weaknesses. Some psychiatrists also do neuro-electrophysiological testing which may help substantiate the diagnosis in confusing cases.

It is very important that the psychiatrist excludes other conditions that may mimic ADD. Problems such as depression (sadness, low self-esteem, withdrawn behaviour), mania (euphoria, over-activity, risk-taking), and obsessive-compulsive disorder, need to be excluded. Some of these are similar to ADD, but the treatment is different.

Treatment of residual ADD

Individuals with residual ADD often have difficulties in a number of areas of their lives. Gaining insight into their problem makes a big difference to their ability to cope with these difficulties. Understanding that the problems arise from ADD often makes it easier for the individual's partner and other members of the family to cope as well. The first step in treatment, therefore, is a proper explanation of the nature of residual ADD and how it affects the person's functioning.

Some adults with ADD require nothing more than this kind of explanation. However, many will need help in the form of medication and counselling.

Medication plays a vital role in helping a person with residual ADD. The adult brain responds just as well as the child's brain to medications used for ADD. Often the doses needed during adulthood are proportionately smaller than those needed for children. For example, an adult may need to take no more Ritalin (methylphenidate) or dexamphetamine per day than a primary school child, despite being considerably heavier.

An adult will need to administer the medication himself, and so issues relating to abuse of these medicines must be understood. With proper controls over the dispensing of medicines such as Ritalin and dexamphetamine, problems with addiction should not occur. The doses of these medicines used in ADD are extremely small, and do not result in any change in mood that would encourage addiction.

All of the medicines used for children with ADD can be used in adulthood. Anti-depressant medication may be very useful in adults with ADD who also have depression. In such cases, higher doses of these medicines are used to obtain an anti-depressant effect.

Individual or group therapy can also be very helpful for adults with ADD. In many cases family therapy or marital guidance will also be helpful. Adults with ADD commonly need help in finding ways of resolving inter-personal conflicts and in addressing marital, family, and occupational problems. Methods for anger control, treatment of addiction, improving self-esteem and refining inter-personal skills are very useful.

Because of the organisational difficulties experienced by adults with residual ADD, the teaching of time management and self-organisational skills is very helpful. Cognitive therapy, where the adult learns how to control thought patterns, is very successful in well-motivated adults with ADD. Social problem-solving and stress reduction can be taught through counselling and role-playing. Group meetings can be helpful, and also provide mutual support and an opportunity to exchange ideas on managing common problems.

Treatment of secondary problems

Many adults with residual ADD have problems with basic academic skills that date from their school days. These may be present even if the ADD difficulties have resolved. There are many ways in which an adult with such difficulties can take steps to overcome them.

It is important to use the aids that are available. If attending lectures, a tape recorder can be used. If difficulties are experienced in taking notes, a friend may be prepared to use carbon paper or make a photocopy of his notes. A computer program may be used to check spelling. An electric typewriter or computer can be used to help produce work that is legible and well presented. For those who are better at typing than writing, there are portable computers and digital diaries. Calculators are portable and have made arithmetic calculations easy for everyone. Spelling dictionaries, both electronic and in book form, are helpful for adults who have spelling difficulties.

For those who have to take examinations, it is usually possible to arrange for allowances to be made for difficulties with reading or writing. It may be necessary to have a letter from a doctor or psychologist to obtain permission to use aids such as a typewriter, scribe, tape recorder or spelling dictionary.

Those who continue to have difficulties with reading may benefit from 'talking books' (recordings of book readings), which are available from many libraries. Some libraries have books written for adults that are easy to read.

Adults who have difficulty with reading or writing should not be embarrassed to ask others to fill in forms for them. Many adults with good literacy skills experience difficulty with forms. Similarly, when taking messages, there is no reason to be embarrassed about asking to have things repeated or spelt out.

If an adult with ADD is undertaking further training, she should inform her lecturers or teachers about her condition, in order that allowances can be made for her difficulties. Most universities have special provisions for the enrolment of people with disability and adults with ADD often qualify for these.

Summary points

- In the majority of children with ADD, difficulties decrease during late adolescence.
- In approximately 20 per cent of children with ADD, the improvement in the late teenage years is so marked that their difficulties can be regarded as having completely resolved.
- Approximately 60 per cent of children with ADD will have mild residual ADD in adulthood. Individuals with mild

residual ADD are not usually hampered by their condition. Some may even turn some of their 'difficulties' into advantages.

- In approximately 20 per cent of children with ADD, severe difficulties persist into adulthood. This hampers their family life and work.
- Many adults who had ADD during childhood will also have secondary problems that arose because of their childhood problems. For example, their ADD may have resulted in failure to attain adequate academic skills, or may have undermined their self-esteem.
- The features of residual ADD include:
  difficulty completing projects
  procrastination
  tackling too many projects at once
  great difficulty starting a task
  easy distractability
  great difficulties with focusing attention
  losing track when reading
  'tuning out' when being spoken to
  impatience
  intolerance of 'red tape'
  restlessness
  intolerance of sedentary activities
  difficulty relaxing
  low frustration tolerance
  frequent temper outbursts
  lack of persistence
  poor organisation
  impulsivity
  tactlessness
  tendency to spend money, change plans, and enact new schemes at short notice
  poor memory
  poor self-appraisal
  mood swings
  tendency to worry needlessly

      sense of impending doom or insecurity

      risk-taking behaviour

- It is very important to exclude conditions that may mimic ADD, such as depression, mania, and obsessive-compulsive disorder. Some of these are similar to ADD, but the treatment is different.
- Gaining insight into their problem makes a big difference to adults with residual ADD. Understanding the cause of the problems makes it easier for the individual's partner and other members of the family to cope.
- Some adults with ADD require nothing more than this sort of explanation. However, many will need help in the form of medication and counselling.
- Medication plays a vital role in helping residual ADD. The adult brain responds just as well as the child's brain to medications used for ADD.
- Individual or group therapy can be very helpful for adults with ADD. In many cases, family therapy or marital guidance will also be helpful.
- Many adults with residual ADD have secondary problems with basic academic skills that date from their school days. These may be present even if the ADD difficulties have resolved. There are many measures an adult with such difficulties can take to overcome them.

Conclusion

All parents want their children to fulfil their academic potential, to be socially successful, and to be well adjusted emotionally. Tragically, many intelligent children fail in one or more of these areas. Although there are a number of reasons why this may happen, many do so because they have ADD.

The best management of ADD is based on early and accurate diagnosis, as outlined in this book. From this diagnostic process an individualised, multi-modal treatment plan can be developed for each child with the condition.

There is no doubt that more and more children with ADD are receiving appropriate diagnosis and treatment. But the task of ensuring that all children with this condition benefit from a modern approach to their difficulties is far from complete. To ensure that this occurs, a wide-spread change in attitudes to children with behavioural, learning, and emotional difficulties is needed. We will need to move away from automatically blaming children and their families for children's learning and behavioural difficulties. We will need to understand that the brain is the organ of learning, of self-esteem, of behaviour, and of emotion. We will need to be open to the possibility that an immaturity of brain function may be the cause of many children's difficulties. We will need to treat

ADD with the same conviction that we presently treat conditions such as asthma and diabetes. With such changes, many more children will be able to look forward to a future of happiness and fulfilment.

Useful addresses

Australia

New South Wales

ADD SUPPORT GROUP SYDNEY
PO Box 200
Baulkham Hills NSW 2153
Telephone (02) 894-0329 [(02) 9894 0329]

Victoria

GEELONG ADDSUP
PO Box 158
Geelong Vic 3220

Queensland

ADD NORTHSIDE SUPPORT GROUP
PO Box 159
Burpengary Qld 4505
Telephone (07) 495-5105 [(07) 5495 5105]

South Australia

ADDSA
Neurological Resource Centre
37 Woodville Road
Woodville SA 5011
Telephone (08) 268-6222 [(08) 8268 6222]

Western Australia

LADS
Chidley Education Centre
Mosman Park WA 6012
Telephone (09) 385-1065 [(08) 9385 1065]

Australian Capital Territory

CANBERRA/QUEANBEYAN ADD SUPPORT GROUP INC
PO Box 53
Duffy ACT 2611
Telephone (06) 290-1984 [(02) 6290 1984]

Tasmania

ADD SUPPORT GROUP TASMANIA
PO Box 514
Ulverstone Tas 7315
Telephone (004) 293-240 [(03) 6429 3240]

Northern Territory

DARWIN ADD SUPPORT GROUP
PO Box 85
Parap NT 0820
Telephone (089) 812-444 [(08) 8981 2444]

United States of America

CH.A.D.D. (Children With Attention Deficit Disorders)
Suite 185, 1857 North Pine Island Road
Plantation
Florida FL 33322
Telephone (305) 857-3700

For books and videos

A.D.D. WareHouse
300 Northwest 70th Avenue
Suite 102
Plantation
Florida FL 33317
Fax 1 305 792 8545

Index